CATCHING
THE CROWN

The Source for Pageant Competition

LU PARKER
MISS USA 1994®

FOREWORD by BOB GOEN
Host, Entertainment Tonight

Requests to the Publisher for permission should be addressed to:
Parker Productions
P.O. Box 6921
San Antonio, Texas 78209

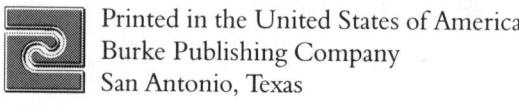

Printed in the United States of America
Burke Publishing Company
San Antonio, Texas

For Mom, Dad & my brother Bill

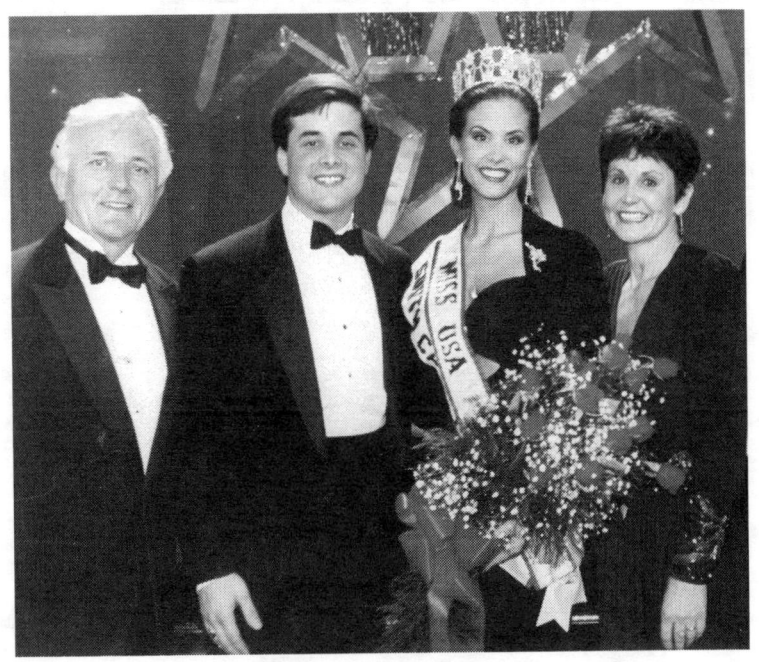

*With my family on stage, minutes after being
crowned Miss USA 1994.*®

ACKNOWLEDGEMENTS

The process of writing this book hasn't been an easy road by any means, but the unbelievable amount of support I received, and continue to receive from my family, friends, and peers has made the journey worthwhile.

Catching the Crown would never be possible if not for Ernie Whiten, my former pageant coach. His advice, patience, and encouragement helped me win the titles of Miss South Carolina USA and Miss USA 1994.® Ernie spent hours, days and weeks by my side. He taught me nearly everything I know about pageant competition. Ernie, thank you for seeing my potential.

It would be impossible to name everyone who has helped me throughout the writing process. You know who you are, and I am grateful everyday our paths crossed. I send special thanks to my brother Bill and to my friends Heather and Bates.

To the Miss Universe Organization, I will always remember an indescribable year with the "family." My experiences with all of you, especially the laughter with Dolores, Marty and Gail, will always be a part of the memories.

The people of South Carolina deserve acknowledgement for their support during and after my pageant competition. Thank you for welcoming me home in such a warm manner.

And to my mentor Ben Mankiewicz, thank you for sharing your advice, and allowing me to share my soul with you.

LU PARKER

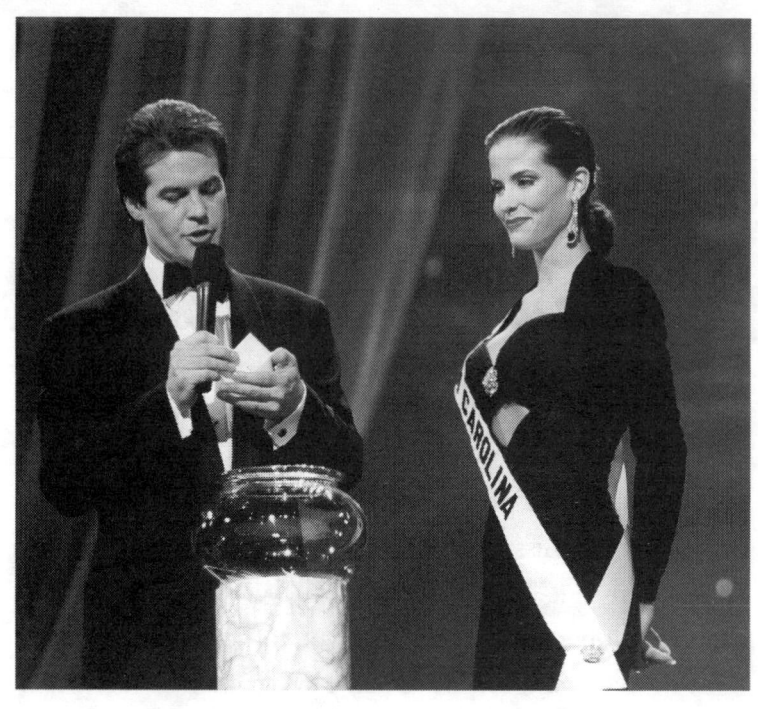

With Bob Goen at the 1994 Miss USA®
pageant right before my top six question.

FOREWORD

I remember my first time hosting the Miss USA Pageant in 1994. With a worldwide television audience of over three million, I knew it was going to be a daunting experience, and to be honest with you, I was a little uneasy about it. But, I thought, "I can't be nervous, because these contestants will need me to calm them down." And, in most cases, that was true, but for one exception. There was one young woman who seemed so poised, so confident, and so together, I felt like leaning on her for strength. That woman was Miss South Carolina USA, Lu Parker. When she walked onto the stage, you just knew there was something special about her. And, when those of us behind the scenes took our straw poll to pick our favorites, Lu was the only unanimous choice.

Chances are, Lu didn't have all the information found in this book at her disposal back then, but now she has put all of her experience and hard-earned knowledge to work for you. What she knows instinctively, and what she learned during her glamorous, yet demanding reign as Miss USA 1994 can help make your journey through the pageant process a memorable one. Your pageant experience should be a highlight in your life. Let **Catching the Crown** show you how to shine!

BOB GOEN
Host, Entertainment Tonight

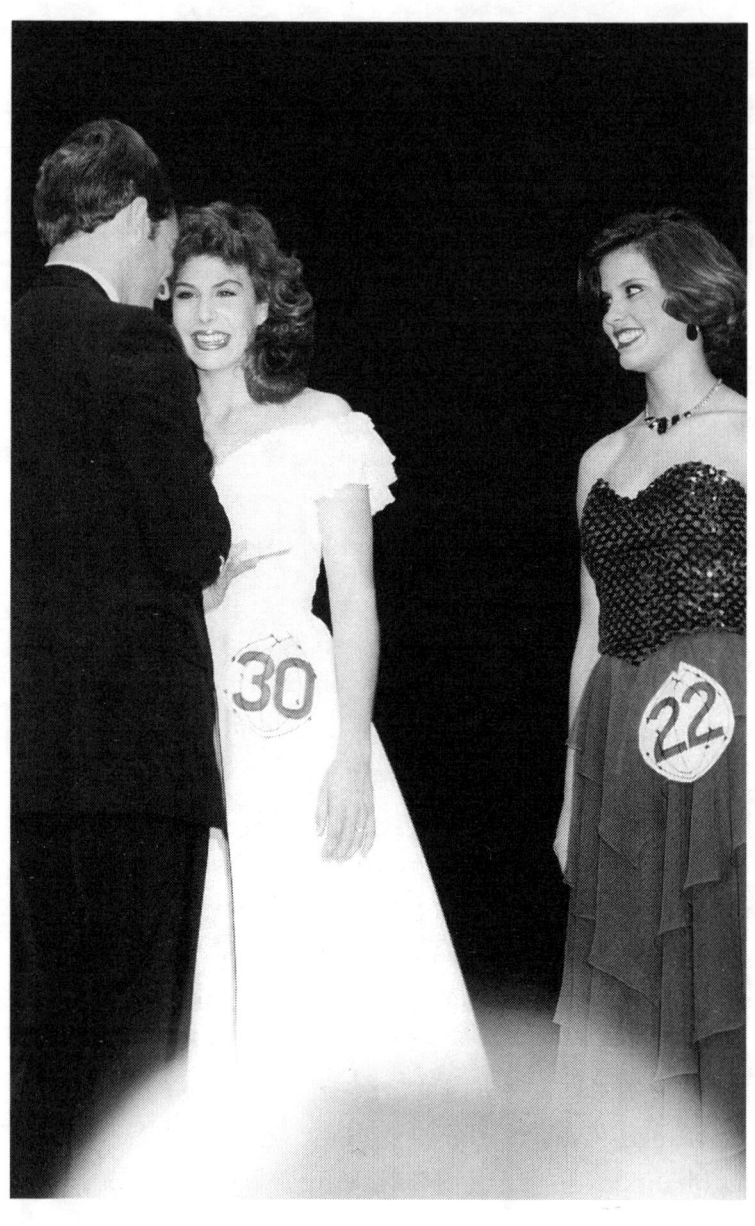

With Gina Tolleson-Thicke, Miss World 1991, in 1983 during the Miss South Carolina Teen USA® pageant.

PREFACE

Why I wrote this book

When I competed in the Miss South Carolina USA® the Miss USA® and the Miss Universe® pageants, there were no books available to help guide and prepare me for the competitions.

I want to introduce the life of pageants to the general public in hopes everyone can find the beauty and worthwhile in them.

I want to share with all of you the wonderful life-changing times I experienced during my pageant years.

When you think of a pageant, you probably think big hair and glittery gowns. You're entitled to your imagination and your opinion, but if you've ever been involved with a pageant, you know it's much more. It's a lot of work, and the delegates diligently prepare for competition. If people took the time to look behind the scenes, they might be pleasantly surprised by what they actually find. I hope the information in **Catching the Crown** will help bring the level of understanding about pageants to a higher degree of respect and appreciation.

To summarize a little about where all this began for me, I will take you back to my first experiences with pageants, and how they evolved. In 1982, as a high school freshman, I competed in my school pageant and luckily won. Then, in 1983, I competed in the South Carolina Teen USA® pageant, placing first runner-up. I entered again in 1984, not placing at all. Honestly, I never thought I would compete in pageants again. I completed high school, college, and then earned my master's degree, and went on to teach high school.

In June 1993, I received a letter from the South Carolina USA pageant office, and when I read it, something told me to "Go for it!" I had nothing to lose (except weight), so I began preparing, and I'm happy I did! All it takes is commitment and tons of work.

No matter who you are: a young person thinking of competing in a pageant, the mother of an interested child, a pageant coach, or a pageant director, I want you to read this book with an open-mind. Use it to enhance and improve performance or just to understand pageants a little more. Please realize these ideas and suggestions aren't written in stone. They're an accumulation of years of experience stemming from the education I received from my friend and coach Ernie Whiten, advice from other winners, from my own research, and even more from personal experiences when I was involved with the **Miss South Carolina USA,**® **Miss USA,**® and **Miss Universe**® pageants. I hope this book is a joy for you to read, and may it help your dreams come true!

CONTENTS

"Destiny is not a matter of chance, it is a matter of choice; it is not a thing to be waited for, it is a thing to be achieved."

– WILLIAM JENNINGS BRYAN .

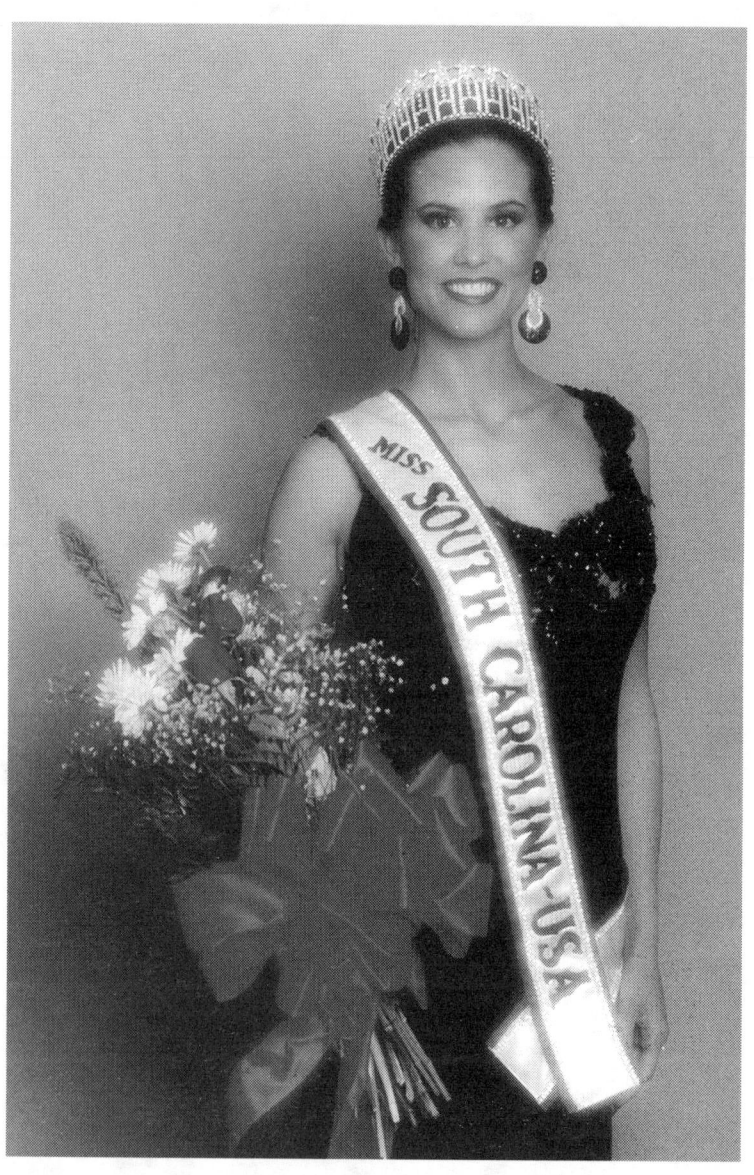

My official picture for the Miss South Carolina USA® pageant.

ARE PAGEANTS FOR YOU?

"Do what you love and the rest will come."
— Unknown

Are you right for pageants?

If you had asked me at age twelve if I were interested in pageants, I would have said "No way!" I was more interested in motorcycles and horses, but as I grew older, I realized pageants might be worth checking out. Pageants aren't for all girls, and that's okay! The burning desire may not be there, and that's okay too! You will know when the opportunity arises if you want to compete. As a matter of fact, if you are reading this book, either you or someone you know is interested in learning more about pageant life. Well, guess what? You've come to the right place!

So, are you right for pageants?

Are you interested in improving yourself?

Are you interested in traveling?

Do you want to help people?

If you answered "Yes" to the above questions, you can compete in a pageant. You may be on your way to **Catching a Crown**!

How to get started

The first thing to do is commit yourself to the task at hand. Is it something you really want to do? It takes a lot of work and dedication to go all the way. If you don't already know which pageant you want to compete in, you should do research. The internet is a great place to get started. Really put some time into this part, because if you were to win, you'll be an employee of a company for a least a year. It's serious business. When you've made the commitment to yourself, and you decide on a particular pageant, then the *fun* and *work* begins!

How much does it cost?

Each pageant is going to be different depending on what's needed for competition expenses, travel time, and entry fee, but if you're truly committed and willing to work, you can compete. When I decided to compete in the Miss South Carolina USA® pageant, I had just finished borrowing close to $15,000 in graduate school loans. I had to pay all my living expenses, and I was teaching high school, which doesn't pay much. I told myself I could find a way to do it all.

THE MAIN COSTS

- Entry fee
- Evening gown
- Swimsuit
- Interview suit
- Pageant coach (optional)
- Physical trainer (optional)

A lot of people think you need to have the most expensive dress, or the best looking wardrobe to win a beauty contest. It's not true. The judges want someone warm, communicative and sincere, not simply a pretty girl in an overpriced dress.

Still, wardrobe is definitely a cost factor. Also, pageants often require you to pay an entry fee at the local and state level. The entry fee helps the state directors pay for overhead costs, and it's how they make a profit. Remember, pageants are serious business. Besides these costs, there's not much more you have to spend unless you decide to hire a pageant coach, or a physical trainer.

Sponsors

After your application and pictures are submitted, most state level pageants offer a sponsor section where you can ask friends, businesses and the public for monetary help. It never hurts to have help in this area, because as I said, competing in a pageant can be very expensive. Most directors offer a package where you can sell advertisements for the pageant program to earn money to pay your expenses, or to use towards your entry fee.

Some delegates have their family sponsor them. That way, your family can put a personal message in the advertisement. Businesses can also write a personal message in their advertisement. None of

SELLING ADS

Example: You sell one full page for the program at $200. Your ad will run in the program and you will usually receive 50% of the earnings. You will earn $100 for your work.

this is necessary if you have the money, but I found it wasn't too difficult to find sponsors, and the extra money helped a lot. Remember, the judges look at the program, so it may help to have your name and picture on more than one page in the program.

Going out in the public and speaking with strangers is great for your self-esteem. It also improves your ability to communicate. The more often you're faced with approaching people you don't know, the more comfortable you'll be during the pageant. The process of selling advertisements will only help you to prepare for the interview segment. Look at it as practice.

Below is an example of a way to approach a business about advertisements. You'll have to modify it depending on the business and situation.

EXAMPLE
Use on the telephone or in a letter.

Hi. My name is____, and I am planning to compete in Miss____ on (date of pageant). To help me with the costs of competing, I am selling advertisement space for the pageant program. Since your business caters to women, I thought it would be great for your business to advertise in the program. May I come by to speak with you to see if you would be interested in buying an advertisement for the pageant program book? I would really appreciate your support.

★ **REMEMBER:** *If you write a letter, be sure to include your phone number so they can get in touch with you.*

Most pageants offer marketing strategies, or will provide data on the number of people the advertisement is projected to reach. Business owners will want to know the numbers. Having them at your disposal will enable you to sell more effectively. Always start with businesses you know.

Be able to sell the pageant system and what it offers individuals, contestants, or a community. Most importantly, sell them on promoting you as the best candidate for the title. Sell yourself! Always remember to send people a thank you note for their support and time.

BUSINESSES

- Clothing boutiques
- Pageant stores
- Banks
- Chiropractors
- Hairdressers
- Nail salons
- TV and radio stations

What are judges looking for?

Judging isn't an easy task. The judges are usually volunteers, and they aren't paid for their time. Many consider being selected an honor. Remember, they're the people who put the crown on your head.

Typically, you're judged on a preliminary and final level. Before the competitions, judges are often briefed in the following areas:

★ **Evening gown Competition:** They're advised to judge each delegate on how she carries herself on stage rather than judging her gown.

★ **Swimsuit Competition:** They're asked not to judge solely on the body, but how the delegate presents herself and carries herself in the swimsuit.

★ **Interview Competition:** The judges are briefed on what's appropriate to talk about and what's inappropriate during the interview. In all likelihood, the judges will shy away from controversial topics like religion, or politics.

★ **Talent Competition:** Because each delegate will present her talent in various ways, the judges are looking for execution on an individual basis. They shouldn't compare one delegate's talent to the next, but should judge each delegate on her timing, strength, emotion, and overall execution.

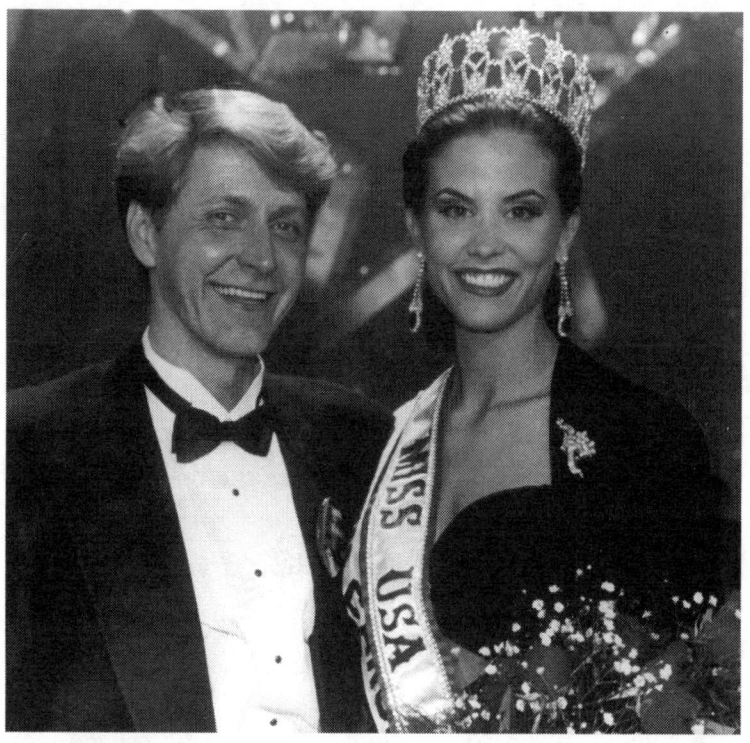

With Ernie Whiten (pageant coach), after I was crowned.

★ **NOTE:** *As the reigning Miss USA 1994,® I spoke with the judges who judged the 1995 Miss USA pageant. I reminded them they only had a limited time to really know the delegates, so make sure they found a young lady who not only had the "gift of the gab," but someone who was truly genuine, compassionate, and most of all "real."*

If you try to trick them with a false demeanor, they'll be able to read it 99% of the time. They're looking for someone genuine. I describe this as getting "good vibes." You want them to connect with you.

Coaches

Pageant coaches, consultants, and advisors are in the business of molding potential delegates. If you can afford this kind of service, and you know of someone with a good reputation, then I recommend you hire one. Again, they aren't necessary to win a contest, but they're great if you can afford it.

Each pageant coach is different, and will have varying opinions, methods of training, and costs. If they've been involved with pageants, they can help you with decisions and with fine-tuning details. You shouldn't feel obligated at any point to continue working with a coach if you decide you're uncomfortable. Be wary if someone asks you to sign a contract for coaching. You can find out about coaches from pageant offices, pageant magazines, and more importantly by word of mouth. Before hiring a coach, find out their experience with pageants and their success rate.

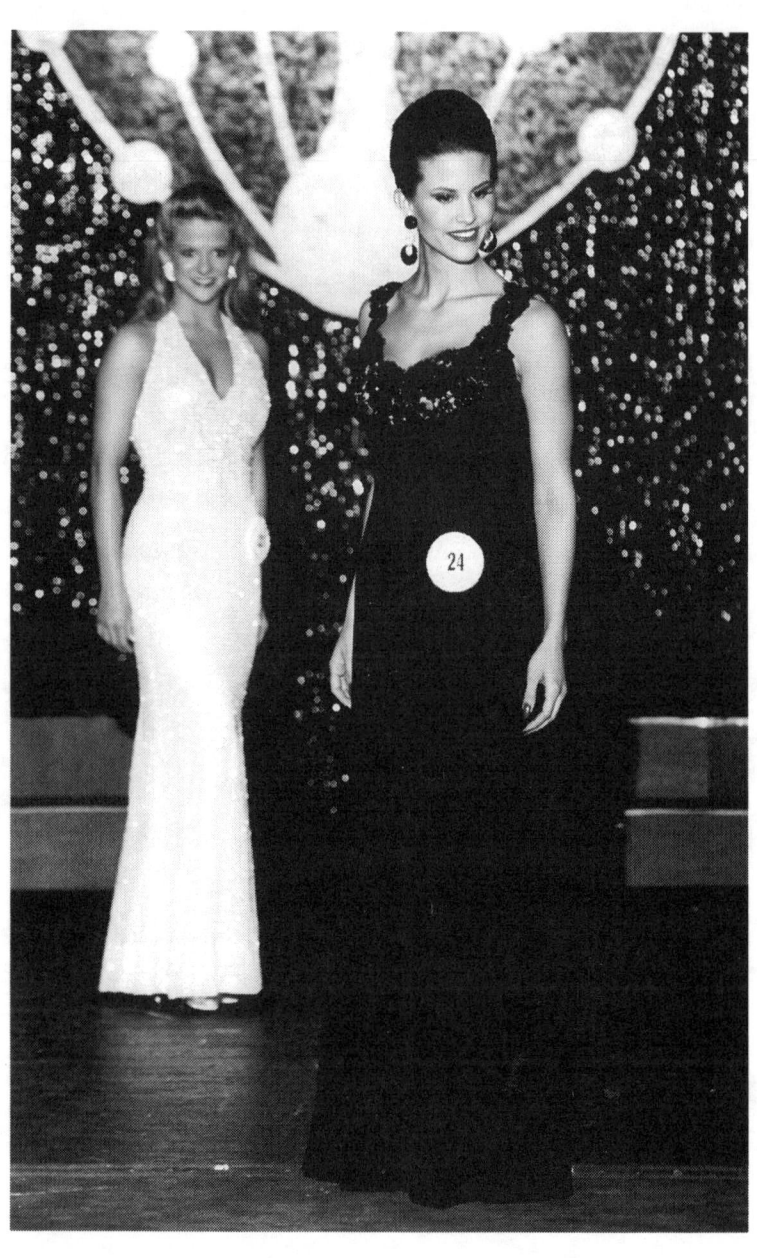

Competing during evening gown competition at the
Miss South Carolina USA® pageant.

YOU'VE DECIDED!

"Aim at the sun, and you may not reach it; but your arrow will fly far higher than if aimed at an object on a level with yourself."
— JOEL HAWES

Mental Attitude

In my opinion, mental attitude is the most important part of preparation. In the early stages of preparation for the Miss South Carolina USA® pageant, I always stepped out of my house with confidence thinking, "I am Miss USA." I never left the house without reminding myself to think that way. I know it sounds silly, but it helps. It kept me focused.

From day one, you must think positively and continually compliment yourself on your progress. Find a way to keep yourself positive throughout the entire process. I can tell you from personal experience as time progresses, and the more exhausted you become, you will doubt yourself at times. That negativity can keep you from reaching your potential, which may cause the judges to doubt you. When I got down, I always looked at the positives around me. I suggest you do the same. Don't dwell on negatives! Ask yourself these questions:

What am I doing to improve myself?
What have I already achieved that I can be proud of?

Believe it! Live it!

Visualize yourself winning. Give up bad habits or situations that get in the way of your goal.

Writing positive affirmations is a great tool for staying positive. **Example:** *"I'm working hard to be my best physically, mentally, and spiritually. I'm the best I can be at this moment. The rewards will be mine for doing so!"*

★ **WRITE YOUR OWN AFFIRMATIONS.** *Do this even if it feels silly.*

_____

_____

_____

_____

_____

_____

_____

A word of warning

In many pageants, there will be delegates more interested in bringing others down rather than elevating themselves. They'll try to use their energy to create self-doubt for other contestants, especially the strong ones. If someone tries to make you feel insignificant, or uncomfortable, then you know it's because you're strong. They see it! Be nice and friendly, but stay focused! Use your energy wisely.

Author Stephen C. Paul once wrote: *"No one has power over you unless you give it to them."*

From the beginning of competition, there will be many beautiful young women with spectacular figures wearing gorgeous gowns, but you absolutely can't concern yourself with what other women may or may not have. If you do, you'll ruin your concentration. Focus on what you have to offer! I had to do it, and it was never easy. I found if I thought only of what positive things I brought to the table, I could ignore the attributes of the other delegates.

Hair

Aren't we always debating how to wear our hair? What a pain! Well, guess what? It's another competition decision you have to make.

Since the judges only have a limited time to see you before they crown you the winner, you want them to automatically recognize

> **TIPS**
> • Keep your hair simple.
> • Keep the ends of your hair trimmed every 4 to 6 weeks to prevent split ends.
> • Condition your hair for shine. There's a lot of wear and tear on your hair during pageants.

you when they see you. There should be no doubt. Therefore, it may be a good idea to wear your hair the same way through all competitions.

Also, make sure your hairstyle is complimentary to your face. You communicate with your eyes, so don't hide them. Your hair should be a part of your overall image. It should never distract from you.

Time is another factor to consider. Don't settle on a style that can't be completed in a hurry. If changing styles is suitable for you, be sure to make simple changes. Time between competitions is very short and hectic.

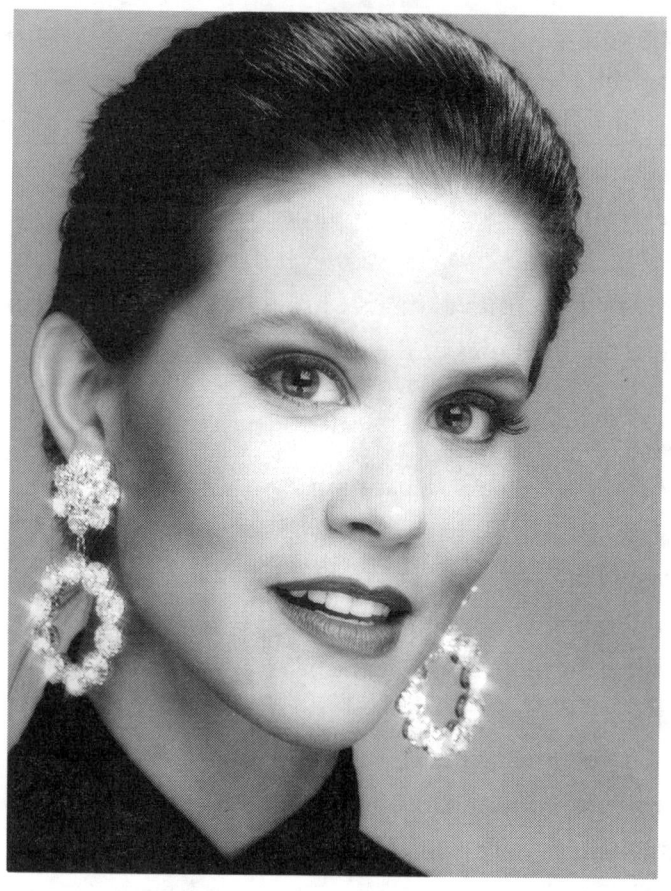

My official picture for the Miss South Carolina USA® pageant.

Skin care

Good skin care is essential for a beautiful complexion throughout life. Make-up, pollution, and oils can clog your skin. Even if you don't wear make-up, you should clean your face at least twice a day.

Basically, it's a simple process and will quickly become

second nature. You should have a quality cleanser, toner, and facial lotion. It's a good idea to exfoliate at least twice a week too. Exfoliating keeps the dirt and dead skin cells free from your face. Remember, drinking water is the secret to beautiful skin.

If you have an acne problem, the best advice I can give is go to a dermatologist. It's well worth the money.

Make-up

If you learn one thing from entering pageants, it's how to apply make-up. I'll never forget how many times I applied make-up during the two weeks I competed for Miss USA, and again for Miss Universe. I can do it in my sleep.

The application of make-up is critical, but if you aren't careful, it can also ruin your look. In this section, let's concentrate on two types of applications: *Day and Stage*

DAY MAKE-UP

Day make-up application is exactly what it implies. Day make-up helps you look beautiful in natural sunlight. I suggest you use the **BASIC 3:** *Foundation, Concealer, and Powder.*

★ **Foundation:** Wear foundation to even skin tone. It's important to make sure your foundation is complimentary to your skin color. Exact skin matches are available from many cosmetic companies. Check shopping malls.

★ **Concealer:** Concealer is used to cover dark circles under your eyes. If you aren't dark under your eyes, just blend foundation. If concealer is overused, it can cause the appearance of lines. Be careful.

★ **Powder:** The powder should be approximately one shade lighter than your base.

★ **Eyeliner:** Brown or black. Pencil and/or liquid works well. Use what makes you comfortable. If you plan to wear false eyelashes, only use liquid eyeliner. Pencils will make the lashes come loose.

★ **Eye shadow:** I suggest neutral colors. This isn't the time to experiment with outrageous colors. Stay natural; this is especially true for teenagers.

★ **Blush:** Keep your blush and lip color in the same color family. *Example*: Pink tone blush with pink tone lips. There's nothing worse than reddish blush with pink tone lips. Yuck!

★ **Lips: Same** as above. Add gloss for shine.

★ **Eyebrows:** The best way to deal with the shape of your eyebrows is to find a reputable salon that can shape them properly. The brow can complete the look, but if you mess this up, it can look horrible. Ask if your eyebrows need to be shaded in with an eyebrow pencil.

★ **REMEMBER:** *The colors on your face should be complimentary with one another. To check for proper application of your make-up, stand by a window with natural sunlight, and use a make-up mirror.*

STAGE MAKE-UP

Stage make-up application is bit different from day make-up. You have to consider intense stage and/or television lighting. If you don't have a proper amount of make-up on, the intense lighting can make you appear pale on camera or stage.

TIPS

- On stage, wear foundation and powder. It makes your skin evenly toned. Feel free to use more coverage.
- False eyelashes are a good idea if you need extra length. However, teenagers shouldn't use false lashes.
- Your blush should be heavier, but again, don't over do it.
- Lips can go a shade or two darker. Definitely use lip liner to shape your lips. The liner should be one shade darker than your lipstick. Add gloss.

Basically, you should wear the same make-up as mentioned earlier, but with a few modifications.

If you feel uncomfortable, consult a make-up artist. Many will customize your make-up with a lesson.

Application & pictures

The application and picture process is extremely important. Some delegates don't realize your picture and your application are all the judges have before they meet you in person. Often, judges will literally pre-judge you based upon your application and picture. That's not a pleasant thought, so take both seriously!

Application

Treat the application as if you were applying for a job. Consider the cash and prizes at each level your salary. Some pageants even offer employment contracts as prizes.

Again, remember your application is how the judges get to know you before they ever meet you. Take care to make sure you invest some quality time with what you write. It's a good idea to make several copies of the original blank application so you can work with it for a while. The entry applica-

TIPS

- Never handwrite the application even if the pageant director says it's okay. Always type!
- Before you send it to the pageant office, get at least two people to proof the final copy of the application.
- Keep a copy of the application for yourself to review *before* and *after* your interview with the judges.
- It's important to know what you wrote on the application. Don't get caught confused about something you put on your application.
- Be honest!

tion will come with one of the original packets you receive from the pageant office.

The space on the application is limited. However, you may be permitted to attach additional sheets. It's best to list all of your honors, accomplishments, volunteer work, talents, and awards in the appropriate categories requested by the application. Be sure to list them in order of most impressive to least impressive, or most unique to least unique. Start the list with the things you feel will catch a judge's eye. If you run out of space, then you know you put the best information in first. Be prepared to talk about whatever you included on the application. Judges often form questions from the topics on your application.

I've inserted a typical application a delegate might fill out when she represents a state for the Miss USA® Pageant. It's very similar to most local, state, and national level applications. Also, I have enclosed my profile page from the 1994 Miss USA® pageant. The judges read this information before they met me.

SAMPLE APPLICATION

Courtesy Miss Universe L.P., LLLP

State _____   Delegate _____

Full name you wish to be called on stage/television and for publicity:

_____

Nickname_____   Why? _____

Hometown (in the state which you are representing) _____

Birthdate _____/_____/_____   Age at last pageant _____

List two major hometown newspapers including address, phone and contact name _____

List brothers and sisters by name and age _____

List your parent's occupations_____

List relatives or ancestors with significant or unusual occupations or achievements_____

Do you have any pets? (Please list type and names.) _____

School(s) currently attending _____

Freshman _____ Sophomore _____ Junior _____ Senior _____

High School_____ Graduated: Yes _____ No _____

Previous College attended _____ Graduated: Yes __ No __

Degree(s) earned _____

Occupation (describe) _____

What is your career ambition? _____

Beyond your career, what would you like to accomplish in the next ten years? _____

If applicable, list any special training you have had (music/drama/art, etc.) _____

Please list your favorites:

Magazine _____

Book or Author _____

Designer _____

Movie Stars (Male, Female) _____

Movie _____

TV Stars (Male, Female) _____

TV Program _____

Recording group or star _____

Sport (as spectator) _____

Sport (as participant) _____

What do you like to do for fun? _____

What world leader would you most like to meet? (why?) _____

If you could live anywhere in the world, where would it be? (why?) _____

_____

_____

If you could live during any historical era, when would it be? (why?)

_____

List three unusual things about yourself or unusual things you have
    done. _____

What person would you most like to meet? (Living, deceased, fictional)
    Why? _____

Have you participated in a pageant prior to winning your title?

_____

_____

If so, please name contest, city, and title (if you won) _____

Do you have a good luck charm? _____   If so, what? _____

What do you believe is the biggest problem facing the world today?

_____

With all the strides women have made politically, educationally and in
    business, is there still a role for beauty pageants in modern society?
    What is it? _____

What do you like most about your state? (Event, tradition, place, etc.)

_____

If you were to be crowned Miss_____, what charitable cause or
    organization would you like to promote or support during your
    reign and why? _____

List your most notable accomplishments. Include awards, scholarships,
    and special achievements. _____

CONFIDENTIAL (for Costuming only)

Height____Weight____Color of Hair____Color of Eyes____Bra & cup___

Waist ____ Hips ____ Hose size (A-D) ____

Shoe size & width ____ Swimsuit size ____

Dress size ____ Hat size ____

SAMPLE PROFILE

Profile of: MISS SOUTH CAROLINA USA

Name: Frances Louise "Lu" Parker

Age: 25

Birthdate: April 16, 1968

Hometown: Charleston

Hair Color: Brown

Eye Color: Hazel

Height: 5'9"

Education: M.A., B.A., The Citadel, The College of Charleston

Occupation: High School English Literature Teacher

Do you have any famous relatives or ancestors? My stepfather is a direct descendant of the Reverend Pierre Robert, who came to South Carolina in 1686 as the second Huguenot minister. He is also a collateral descendant of General Henry Martyn Robert, author of "Robert's Rules of Order," and of General Alexander Lawton, who was a U.S. minister to Austria and a founder of the American Bar Association.

What is your career ambition? To continue my career as an educator while maintaining my position as executive director of the H.A.T.S. (Helping All Teens Survive) Program.

List any special training you have had: I've had nine years of instruction in jazz, tap and ballet, three years of piano lessons, one year of voice, and also public speaking.

What do you like to do in your spare time? I enjoy writing poetry, reading, riding horses, and traveling.

What is your most cherished childhood memory? The memories of playing hide-and-seek in the corn fields with my brother and the family black lab.

If you have learned on thing in life, it is: To believe in yourself wholly, but to realize that without others you are nothing.

What person would you most like to meet? The Secretary of Education, Richard Riley. I'd like to have the opportunity to personally present to him the H.A.T.S. Program in an effort to secure his endorsement and assistance.

Three words that best describe who you are: Influential, Determined and Dedicated.

What made you decide to enter a pageant? Nominations from my peers resulted in my first two pageant competitions. The motivating factor behind my entering the Miss South Carolina USA Pageant resulted from a long term goal to become Miss Universe, which would enable me to become a much needed, highly visible role model for the youth of the world.

What do you like most about your state? My love for South Carolina geographically stems from its versatility. We not only have the beauty of the ocean, we also offer the mystery of the mountains, and the excitement of the cities in between.

Favorite book or author: Edgar Allan Poe, "Education of Little Tree" by Forrest Carter.

Favorite movie: "Beaches"

Favorite movie stars: Jack Nicholson, Glenn Close

Favorite TV program: "60 Minutes"

Favorite TV stars: Dan Rather, Oprah Winfrey

Picture

Your picture can make or break you in some cases. It is imperative you choose a picture representative of you. Here are a few suggestions:

★ *If you're a teenager, never submit a picture that makes you look grown up or too sexy. Look like a teenager.*

★ *Make sure the background of the picture is light enough so you won't fade into the background. For women of color, make sure the background isn't too dark.*

★ *Smile and look natural! Sexy doesn't always work. Confidence always does!*

★ *Never wear a crown or a hat in the picture unless requested to do so.*

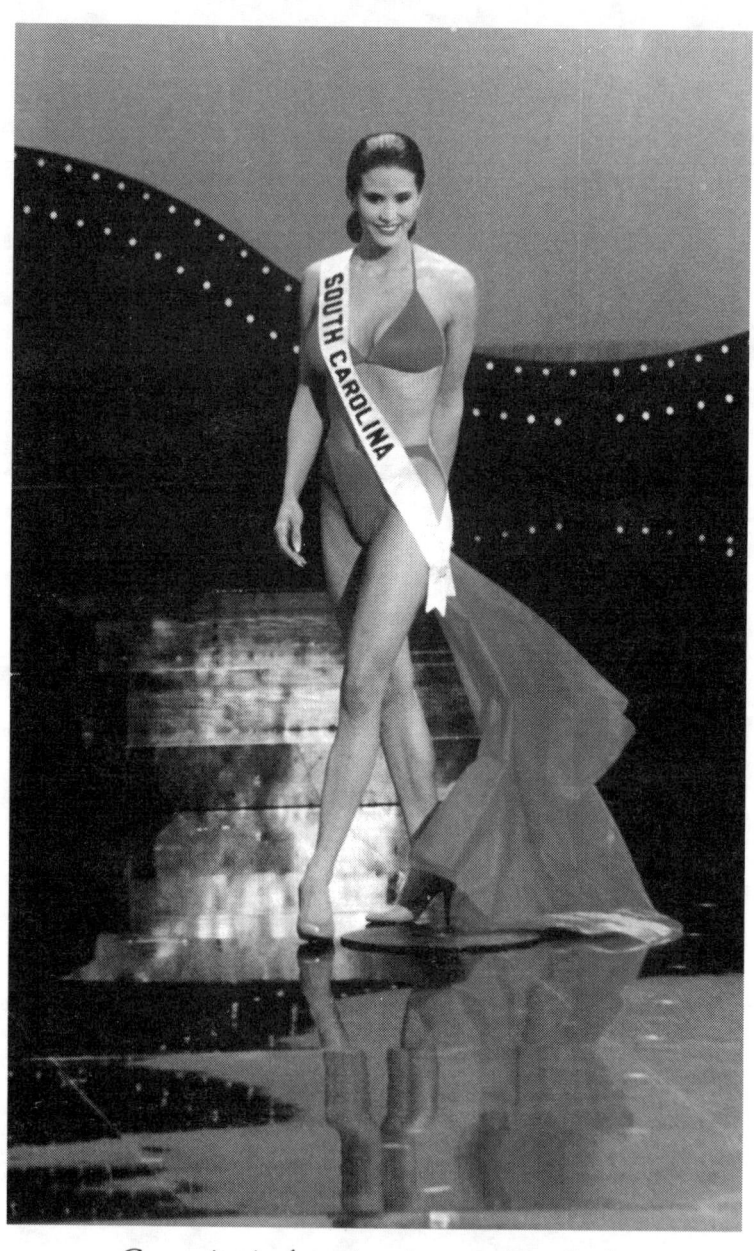

Competing in the swimsuit competition for the
1994 Miss USA® pageant.

COMPETITION
PREPARATION

"I find the great thing in this world is not so much where we stand,
as in what direction we are moving."
— OLIVER WENDELL HOLMES

Pageants normally consist of 3 to 4 areas of competition: INTERVIEW, SWIMSUIT, EVENING GOWN, and in some pageants, TALENT. From the start, you should think about improving yourself mentally, physically, and if needed, begin fine-tuning your talent for competition.

Thoughts on Interview

I especially like this part of competition, and I also believe it is the most important. There are tricks of the trade, so pay close attention here.

In most pageants, you will be required to interview not only on stage, but also with judges individually. For instance, in the Universe system, each judge interviews every delegate alone for four to five minutes. The top three and top six finalists are also asked additional questions on stage during competition. In some pageant systems, the judges are

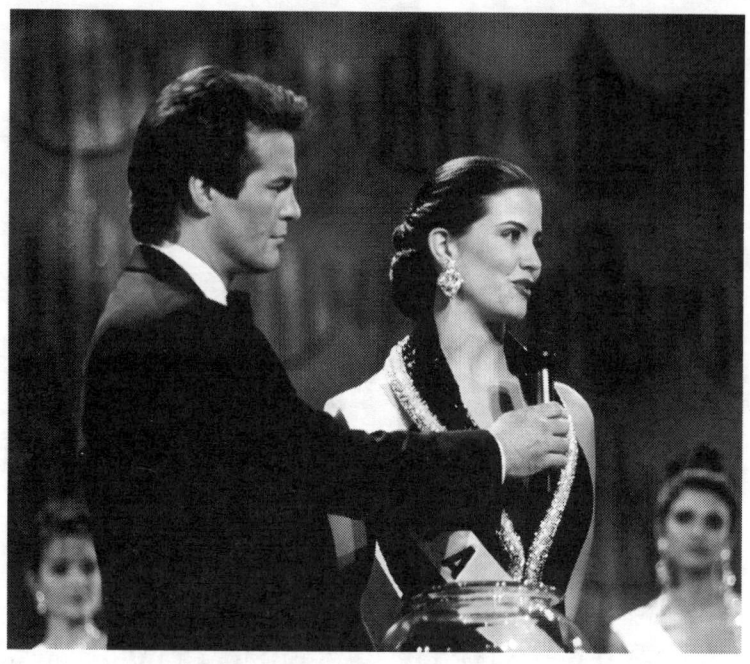

*Bob Goen holds the microphone for me as I answer my top six
question in the 1994 Miss Universe® pageant.*

grouped as a panel. They interview a delegate as a group in
one room.

The most important thing to remember is the judges
aren't there to hurt, embarrass or humiliate you. Whenever delegates, at any pageant, ask for my advice, I tell them
not to forget the judges are human. They're mothers and
fathers. They cry. They laugh. I calmed down before going to an interview by saying to myself *"These judges I'm
about to meet are new friends. I want to get to know them. I want
them to know I'm the best candidate for this job."*

To better prepare for the task of interviewing, it's imperative you constantly interview and talk with strangers until the competition. By keeping yourself out in the public, you'll gain more confidence, develop self-esteem, and become more comfortable meeting people for the first time. The more you keep your mind active, and the more often you speak with strangers, the better you'll do. TALK! TALK! TALK!

If you win the pageant, it will be part of your job to talk with strangers. If you care about people, let it show. Speak to them. Introduce yourself. Shake hands. Look them in the eye. If you can't do this, pageants may not be for you.

When I was preparing for the Miss South Carolina USA® and Miss USA® pageants, I interviewed public officials in Charleston, South Carolina, where I lived. You can start with the chief of police, the mayor, and city officials. Local college professors, doctors, and lawyers are great too. People in these positions are usually very willing to speak with you in person. Call their office and tell them who you are, what you're preparing for, and ask if they would be willing to sit with you for a few minutes. When the meeting is arranged, make a list of at least 10 prepared questions. Also, be prepared to ask them what they would ask in a pageant interview. They will probably share a lot with you about what they would expect from a titleholder.

Although you are conducting the interview, treat the interview as if "pageant judges" are interviewing you. Talking to people we know is easy, but you won't know the judges, so learn to overcome the inevitable fear by talking to strangers. Judges are, once again, just people.

When I was preparing for the Miss USA® pageant, I took

the interviews to a higher level by traveling to Washington, D.C. to speak with officials at nine embassies and with two U.S. senators. When you push yourself, it prepares you even more as a candidate. Always send a handwritten thank you note after the interview.

Current events & questions

Not all pageants test you on your knowledge of current events, but all pageants will, in some way, test your belief system. While I was preparing for competition, I bought index cards, and kept them with me at all times. I recommend you do the same.

Whenever you think of something that might come up in a question, whether it's an article out of the newspaper, or an opinion you agree with from a Sunday morning talk show, write it on one of the index cards. Use a different card for each question. I suggest you keep these cards with you at all times, and refer to them whenever possible. Don't forget to carry them to the pageant, because it helps to fill down time during rehearsals. When I went to the Miss USA® pageant, I had over 100 cards I collected over a five-month period.

Even though I often wanted to chat and laugh with the other delegates, I always reviewed my cards during breaks. You can laugh and chat after you win the crown. I'm not advising you to be rude or mean, but I am saying **STAY FOCUSED**!

Many delegates undermine their chances when they fail to know important information about the county, state, and country they represent. It's embarrassing to see Miss____ unable to name her own governor. Also, know your state tree, bird, and flower. It can't hurt.

During preparation, read the newspaper daily. Set aside a certain amount of time during the day to sit and read the paper thoroughly. When you read something interesting, put it on one of the index cards. When you read the paper or research an issue, take time to stop and think about how you feel about the issue. Ask yourself if you can articulate an opinion on the topic and then validate it. If you can't make a convincing argument, you need to do more research.

Possible questions

In this section, I included some of the sample questions I've collected over the years. When answering the questions for the first time, read the questions and immediately state an opinion on paper as if you were saying it on stage. You want your initial answers to flow freely. Do not judge yourself during this process.

Try to be thoughtful with your answers. These aren't yes or no questions. Expand on them. Always think!

★ Who do you feel has been the most influential woman of all time?

★ What would be your goals and objectives be should you win the title of Miss_____?

★ What do you think is the most critical issue in society today?

★ What would constitute a perfect date, day, husband, child, life for you?

★ What is one interesting thing you would like to share with me today?

★ Why did you decide to be in the pageant?

★ Some people say the eyes are the windows to your soul. If I were to look into your eyes to your soul, what would I see?

★ Who has been the most influential person in your life?

★ If you could be on any television show, which one would you be on and why?

★ If you could be in any movie, which one would it be?

★ If you had 10 seconds to do a commercial for something you truly believed in, what would you say? 30 seconds?

★ Racism still exists in the school systems. What would you do to attempt to change or improve the situation?

★ What are 3 foods that describe you?

★ Do politicians truly reflect the wishes and feelings of the people they represent?

★ What is your favorite part of competition?

★ What is your least favorite part of competition?

★ If you could swap places with one person, who would it be?

★ If you could be any other place, where would it be?

★ What one thing would you change about yourself?

★ What is one thing you would change about the world?

★ Why do you think you should be Miss_____?

★ If you could take a judge on a tour of the state of which you are from, where would you take him/her?

★ If you could put 3 things in a time capsule to be taken out in 100 years, what would you put in the capsule?

★ If you had the power to pass a new law, what would it be?

★ How do you feel about plastic surgery?

★ Who do you feel is the most influential woman in today's society?

★ If you discovered your roommate had somehow secured the questions that would be asked at the pageant, what would you do?

★ If I gave you a six-inch string, what would you do with it?

★ Describe yourself.

★ Describe your career goals.

★ If you could know something about your future, what would it be?

Interview Exercise

Give family and friends a copy of your completed application. Have them ask you potential interview questions while you stand in front of them as if you were on stage. It's very important the person who asks the question not critique the answer. Immediately move to the next question. Record the session to be your own critic. Always remember, the judges will be asking for your opinion, not those of your family and friends.

> **TIP**
>
> When a judge asks you a question, think to yourself: What is the most intelligent way to answer?

Even though I have listed a number of possible questions, I can't stress the next few points enough! Most importantly, you must know who you are, and what has made you the person you are today. Ask yourself these questions, and answer them honestly.

Who am I?
What issues do I feel strongly about?
What are my areas of expertise?
What am I striving for in life?
What is important to me?
What experiences in life have brought me to this point?

If you answered the questions honestly, you're on your way. You'll understand yourself better, and you'll believe in yourself. And that self-confident attitude will come across in the interview section. You don't want rehearsed answers. That's a sure-fire way to a low score, but confident answers score high.

When rehearsing answers in your head, answer in general terms. If you begin answering questions with set answers, you'll only get frustrated and confused on stage and in the private interview. Relax, let the judges see the real you. The mission isn't to memorize an answer, but to figure out how you feel about the issue. The answer will then come naturally from within you.

Interview dress

In most cases, the judges see you in person for the first time during the interview. You're generally allowed to wear whatever you choose, but here are a few suggestions and tips.

When I competed in Miss South Carolina USA® and Miss USA,® and Miss Universe,® I wore a basic black suit. They were figure flattering, but were also simple enough the judges listened to what I was saying instead of what my suit looked like. I also wore very simple jewelry. You want them to remember your eyes, your smile, and your personality, not your clothes.

TIPS

- Wear something professional – a suit, nice dress, or dressy pantsuit. Think of this as a job interview.
- Don't wear sequins.
- Your dress or suit should reflect the specific pageant. **Example:** For a teen pageant, you can dress more stylish. For scholarship pageants, you might decide to dress a little more conservative. For others, like the USA affiliates, you can go more glamorous.
- Don't wear hats.
- Stay away from green outfits when competing. Studies show people sometimes psychologically think of money when they see green. It may sound crazy, but you can't take the chance.
- Be sure to wear day make-up, but don't over do it. Save the stage make-up for competition.

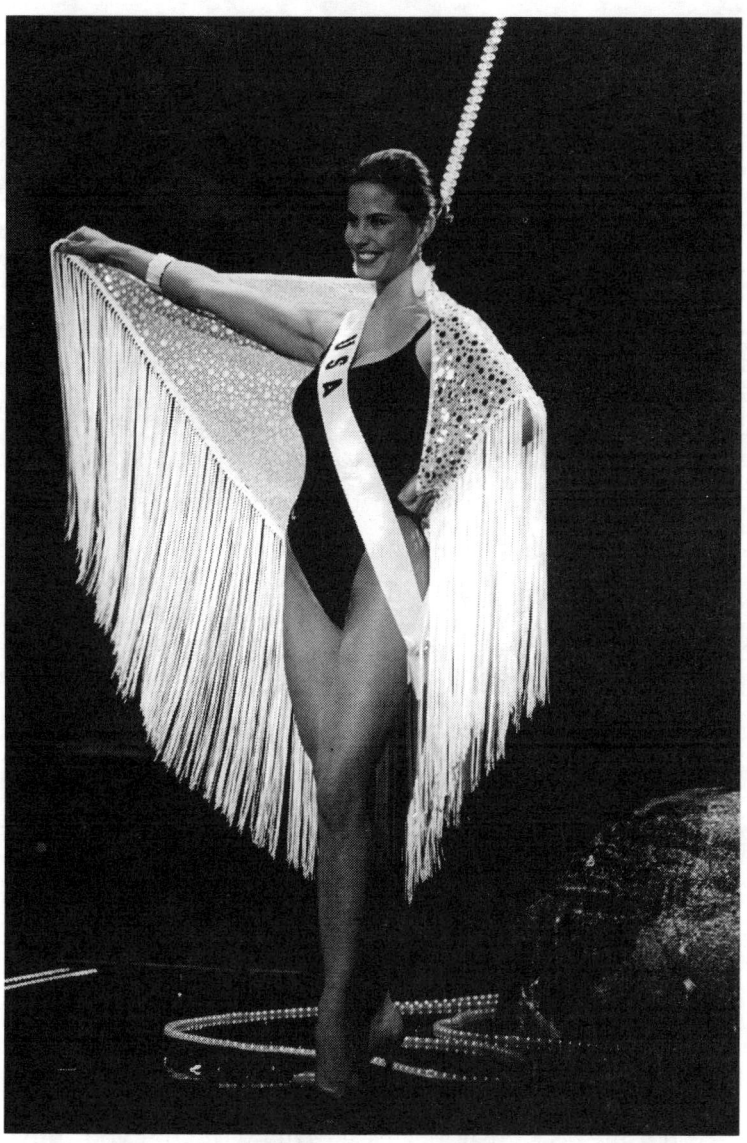

*Competing in the swimsuit competition during the
Miss Universe® pageant.*

Physical preparation

When you begin preparing yourself physically for the competition, you'll definitely need a positive attitude. I know I did! It's not easy work to balance all the facets of preparation, but if you remain focused and organized from the beginning to end, you'll be successful.

Most competitions include a swimsuit or physical fitness section. Because this is such an important part of competition, it's a good idea to analyze your overall look. After you decide what you'd like to improve on and figure out time limitations, set some fitness and appearance goals.

When I decided to compete for the Miss South Carolina USA crown, I sent in my application in August for a December competition. I sat down immediately and decided what I needed to do to be ready for competition. At that time, I felt I needed to lose 10 to 15 pounds. I not only had to increase my physical activity, but I had to become aware of my eating habits. I set small goals and began seeing results immediately.

My life was busy during the time of preparation. I would teach school until 3:00 PM, and then would go to the gym and ride the bike for 90 minutes every day. I also stopped eating sweets and dairy products. The point is, I looked at what needed to be done and I did it. You can too!

It's always a great idea to actually write out your physical goals. It keeps you focused to chart your progression on a daily basis. I called my system the "Goal Record." Every day I kept track of what I ate, how long I exercised, and my weight loss. The "Goal Record" enabled me to visualize my progress on a regular basis. Of course, you have to modify it to fit your needs. You can use the following format as an example. Make one for each day, and be sure to fill it out consistently. Do what works best for you.

GOAL RECORD
This is an example of the one I used back in 1993.
You should modify it to fit your needs.

Date_____

I am starting a fitness and diet program today to get ready for the Miss_____Pageant. (Be specific here.) I have____days to reach my goal. I will work one week at a time. Each week I'm going to see results. I will exercise 6 days a week, and will watch what I eat. This is the beginning of a new lifestyle.

GOALS
★ To get to a size____
★ To lose weight and/or tone so I can win the swimsuit competition.
★ To work one week at a time.
★ To feel good about myself by remaining positive and focused.

NOT ALLOWED
★ Salt
★ Cream or milk
★ Bread
★ Alcohol
★ Pretzels

CHECK LIST
☐ 8 glasses of water
☐ Vitamins
☐ Exercise

Breakfast: _____

Lunch: _____
_____
_____

Snack: _____

Dinner: _____
_____
_____

Total Daily Calories: _____
Weight: _____

Comments: _____
_____
_____

Losing weight

Losing weight doesn't have to mean losing your mind. You can still eat. The best way to lose weight is to eat three to four small healthy meals a day, exercise at least four times a week for at least 30 minutes each day, and drink eight glasses of water a day. If possible, you should speak to a professional, a personal trainer, or a nutritionist about a specific plan.

Unfortunately, when you arrive at the pageant, there will be plenty of food available, and often the pageant events are centered around eating. At the local and state level, you should be okay because the pageants only last about 3 days. But, when

TIPS
- Eat three to four small, low-fat meals a day.
- Exercise 4-5 times a week for at least 30 minutes. Activities like running, walking, swimming, aerobics, cycling, and the stair-climber are great for burning fat.
- Drink at least 8 glasses of water a day.

you compete in a large state, or on the national and international level, beware! You'll be there up to three weeks. You can ruin everything you've achieved. Stick to the routine you've been using, and stay focused!

I used mental games with myself to help get me through the two weeks at the MISS USA® pageant. Each day at lunch, there was always a cake for the delegates. I have a huge sweet tooth, so I constantly fought the urge to eat it. But I succeeded, because I would ask myself, "Do I want a piece of cake, or do I want the car I'll win if I'm crowned Miss USA?" The car always won. I never ate the cake, and I walked away with the car!

Gaining weight

Gaining weight is difficult for women who are naturally thin. When they try to gain weight by eating, the new weight usually goes to one specific area, like the stomach. For some, it's a never-ending battle.

Vitamins

During your busy preparation time, you're going to need energy. Vitamins can help tremendously. Find a quality Multi-Vitamin to take during your months of preparation.

TIPS
- Exercise to tone.
- Don't burn calories by doing cardiovascular exercises like running, walking, and cycling. Instead, get on a weight lifting program to help build muscle. This will give you better definition and bulk.
- Snack throughout the day between your meals.
- Eat before you go to bed.

★ **REMEMBER**: *Caffeine and vitamins don't mix. If taken within two hours of each other, caffeine will often deplete all vitamin resources.*

Sleep

It is imperative you coordinate plenty of sleep with vitamins and physical fitness. Our bodies won't function if we don't sleep properly. You should get at least seven hours of sleep a night, and if your body says you need a nap in the middle of the day, take one. A 20-30 minute nap will give you renewed energy.

Nails

Someone once said, *"A princess is a woman who keeps herself properly groomed all the way to the tips of her fingers."* Your hands often reflect how you care for yourself. I suggest you wear an everyday length during competition. If you decide to color your nails, be sure to keep the color combinations in line with your wardrobe. It's best to choose one color and stick with it so you don't have to be concerned with changing colors during the days of competition. Again, remember your nails shouldn't take away from you and your personality.

Sun exposure

For the swimsuit competition, you'll want to have a slight tan. I found the easiest way to get tan was to use a standing tanning capsule at a salon. It gave me an even tan, and it saved time. Don't wear underwear or a bra in the tanning bed because you'll have tan lines during competition. Also, cover your face during tanning. The first reason is simple: wrinkles! The second, if your face is too tan, your make-up and features will look dark while on stage.

You can always use darker make-up to match your body. You want to have an overall healthy color to your skin, but don't overdo it!

Choosing a swimsuit

Depending on the pageant, there will be swimsuit specifications and requirements. Be sure to check with your local and state directors about swimsuit regulations. Some pageants require a certain style suit. Unless the pageant director tells you otherwise, you should always wear a one piece for local and state level pageants.

Choose a swimsuit complimentary to your skin color and figure. Consultants often say dark colored suits such as black, blue or brown are good for appearing thinner on stage. Bright colors are good too. If you are thin and want to appear larger, experts suggest light colored swimsuits such as white, cream or yellow. Solid colored suits work the best for stage. Stripes and dots can make you appear larger than you are.

When choosing shoes for swimsuit competition, I suggest wearing nude colored heels. The nude color keeps the judge's eyes on you and your figure, rather than your feet. The higher the heel is, the better. Heels make your legs look longer, but be sure you can walk in them without stumbling. If you can't, don't wear them.

Choosing an evening gown

Of course, the evening gown you choose is very important! Not only is this a big part of competition, but it's also

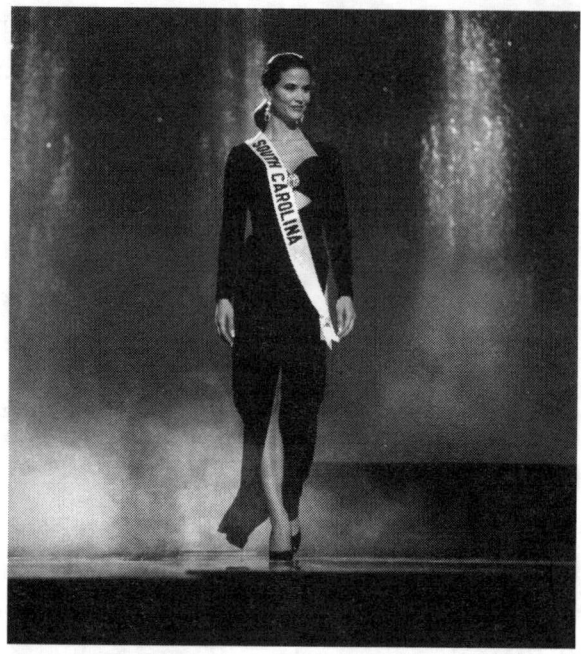

Evening gown competition during the Miss USA® pageant. I received the highest score among the finalists.

TIPS

- The evening gown should definitely be long, not cocktail or three-quarter length.
- Avoid bright colors that distract from your face and figure.
- Both full skirts and slim cut skirts work.
- You may have to walk down stairs in some cases, so be sure you can walk comfortably not only in your dress, but also in your shoes.
- Your shoes should be the same color as your gown.

representative of who you are. Decide if the image you want to portray is conservative, sexy, sophisticated, flashy, or a combination.

Because I was a high school teacher when I competed in the Miss South Carolina USA®, Miss USA® and Miss Universe® pageants, I wanted to go with a sophisticated look

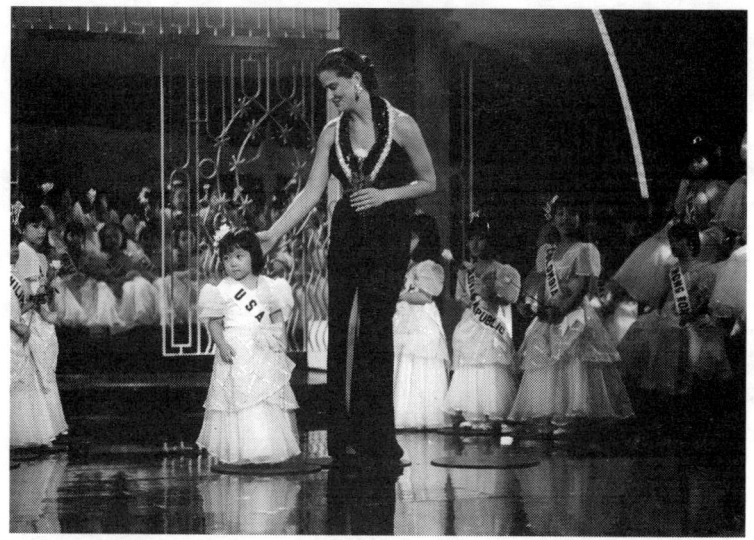

With my adopted Filipino little sister during the evening gown competition at the Miss Universe® pageant.

that wasn't too sexy, but I didn't want to be overly conservative either. In all three pageants, I wore a different black dress.

★ **TEENS REMEMBER:** *You are competing for a teen title. You should look like a teenager. Stay away from sexy.*

Deciding on a talent

The Webster's Dictionary defines **talent** as "a special often creative or artistic aptitude of a person." When you have to compete with a talent, don't shy away! **Get creative!** You can be as innovative as you want. Use any of your hobbies as a talent. Make the judges remember your performance! To do this, you need to prepare thoroughly. Remember, the judges

TIPS

- Make a definite decision on your performance early.
- Practice! Practice! Practice!
- Schedule a talent practice time within your day just as you do for interview preparations.
- Perform on stage as frequently as possible.
- Perform in front of people as often as possible. Ask for input.

want to enjoy your talent. They aren't there to criticize you.

While you want to be as creative as possible, you also need to stay within the required time period. Most pageants run on a tight schedule, so there will be a set time for your performance. Be sure to ask your pageant director what's required.

Packing

If you plan ahead and stay organized, packing can be easy. It's important to list all the outfits you plan to take with you to the pageant. If you don't, I guarantee, you'll leave something behind. When you're preparing to pack for a pageant, try to do it slowly in a 2 to 3 day period instead of waiting until the last minute. It takes much longer than you might expect.

★ NOTE: *The judges only see you during the interview, swimsuit, evening gown, and/or talent competitions. If once or twice, you have to repeat your outfit for a luncheon or benefit, it's truly okay! Believe me! I did it many times. It has nothing to do with who wins. Plus, it will help you maintain your sanity and your budget.*

COMPETITION CLOTHING

☐ Sash *(if needed)*
☐ Swimsuit *(if needed)*
☐ Swimsuit shoes *(neutral color)*

★ NOTE: *No jewelry should be worn during swimsuit competition*

☐ Interview outfit
☐ Interview shoes
☐ Accessories

☐ State costume
☐ State gift *(if needed)*

☐ Talent costume *(if needed)*
☐ Accessories
☐ Shoes
☐ Props

☐ Evening gown
☐ Evening gown shoes
☐ Accessories

GENERAL CLOTHING

☐ Registration/Arrival outfit
☐ Shoes
☐ Accessories

☐ Rehearsal clothes
☐ Shoes (very comfortable)
☐ Non-competition swimsuit and cover

★ NOTE: *Carry your competition shoes with you to rehearsals so you can practice walking on stage and on stairs during the rehearsal breaks.*

Daytime Outfits
(Depending on the weather)

☐ Slacks with top
☐ Skirt with top

☐ Sundress

★ NOTE: *The number of outfits depends on the length of the trip.*

☐ Cocktail dresses

★ NOTE: *Have you packed accessories and shoes for each outfit? Try to use the same shoes for as many outfits as possible.*

Accessories

- ☐ Evening purse
- ☐ Daytime purse
- ☐ Tote/gym bag
- ☐ Hats *(if needed)*
- ☐ Gloves *(if needed)*
- ☐ Rainwear
- ☐ Evening shawl
- ☐ Sweater or jacket for rehearsals *(It's often cold in auditoriums.)*

Lingerie

- ☐ Bras: ____ white ____ black ____ strapless
- ☐ Panties *(# depends on the length of the trip)*
- ☐ Slips *(if needed)*
- ☐ Nylons *(bring extras and assorted colors)*
- ☐ Nightgown
- ☐ Robe *(great to use in the dressing room during competition)*

Grooming

- ☐ Eyeglasses/Contact lens supplies *(if needed)*
- ☐ Brush/comb
- ☐ Shampoo/Conditioner
- ☐ Styling mousse or gel
- ☐ Hair dryer
- ☐ Curlers *(if needed)*
- ☐ Hairpieces *(if needed)*
- ☐ Make-up mirror *(helps in the dressing room)*
- ☐ Cosmetics
- ☐ Skin-care products
- ☐ Lotion
- ☐ Cotton balls/Q-tips
- ☐ Toothbrush/toothpaste/ mints

★ **NOTE:** *Do not take gum. It's unattractive. Enough said.*

- ☐ Deodorant
- ☐ Manicure items
- ☐ Perfume
- ☐ Tampons
- ☐ Sunscreen
- ☐ Razor

Miscellaneous Items

- ☐ Airline ticket *(if needed)*
- ☐ Spending money

★ **NOTE:** *Meals are provided for delegates at most pageant competitions.*

- [ ] Adapter plugs *(international travel)*
- [ ] Detergent *(for small cleanings)*
- [ ] Camera/film
- [ ] Batteries
- [ ] Walkman/tapes/CD's
- [ ] Umbrella
- [ ] Sunglasses
- [ ] Travel iron
- [ ] Alarm clock
- [ ] Pens
- [ ] Journal-Address book/ stationery/stamps
- [ ] Extra bag for miscellaneous gifts you may receive

Note: *Emergency care is often provided at pageants.*

- [ ] Sewing kit *(small)*
- [ ] Safety and straight pins
- [ ] Eye drops *(good for early mornings)*
- [ ] Prescription medicine
- [ ] Band-Aids
- [ ] Aspirin
- [ ] Vitamins

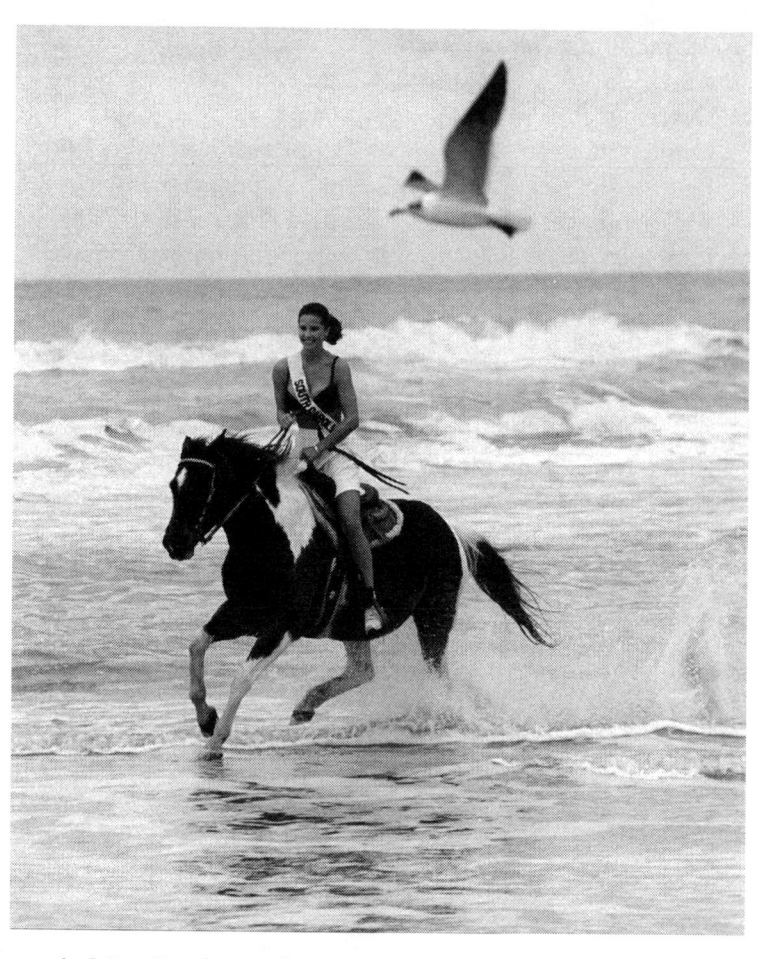

As Miss South Carolina at the 1994 Miss USA® pageant, during a promotional shoot. Newspapers around the country carried the Associated Press photograph.

AT THE PAGEANT

"He knows the water best who has waded through it."
— DANISH PROVERB

What to expect

The key word is **excitement!** You ought to be thrilled competing for a prestigious title, and you have excited people surrounding you. The pageant director and the staff have all worked hard to make the events special for you and the other delegates. Though your nerves may be frayed at the beginning, remember, this is a great opportunity. **Relax! Stay focused & positive!**

On the local or state level, a director and staff run the pageant. These people welcome your questions and concerns, but it's a good idea to let them introduce and explain all the details before you begin questioning. The same applies for national and international pageants. You are their responsibility during the pageant, so they'll explain in detail what's expected of you during competition.

National and international pageant competition is much larger, and as you might expect, it's a huge business. It includes pageants such as Miss Teen USA,® Miss USA,® Miss Universe,® Miss America, and Miss World. These are professional productions with sponsors, and a significant staff behind the scenes.

Arrival

By this time, you have chosen what you're going to wear on arrival day. Your decision will obviously depend on the weather and the time of year.

If you have an early morning registration, arrive in the city the evening before so you can get a good night's rest. Registration is a time to meet and greet, and the delegates are often introduced to the director and staff. If you're asked to introduce yourself, don't be nervous! Be proud of the preparations you have made! Sometimes parents are allowed to come to registration on the local and state level, but eventually you'll be on your own.

Roommates

At pageants, you'll almost always be paired with a roommate during your stay. I was lucky to have great roommates for the Miss South Carolina USA,® Miss USA,® and Miss Universe® pageants. Dealing with roommates can be stressful, but don't let it get to you. Just be considerate and patient. There's often limited space for clothes, suitcases, and make-up, but if you take each other's feelings and needs into account, your time together will go smoothly.

I think the number one problem with roommates is the telephone. Remember to think of the other girl. Don't hog the phone! She may be trying to sleep, or expecting a call herself. And remember those common

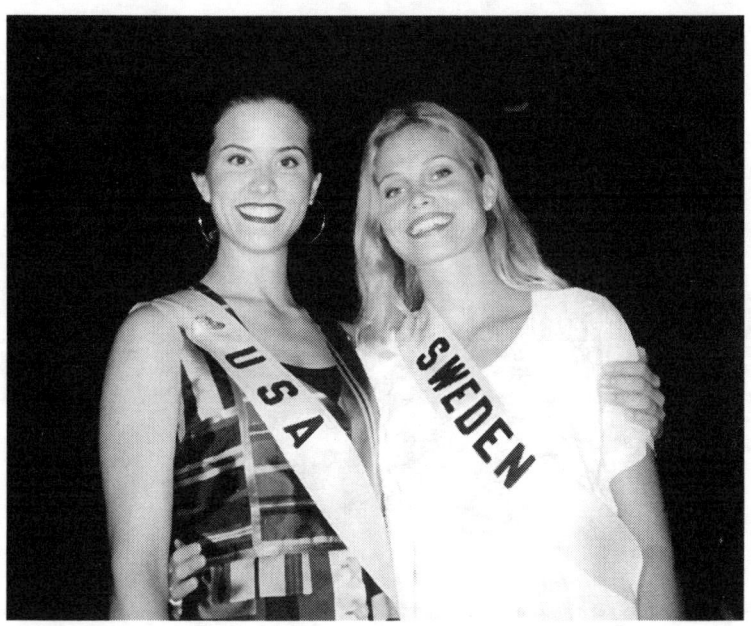

With my roommate, Dominique Forsberg, Miss Sweden, at the Miss Universe® pageant in Manila, Philippines.

courtesies like being quiet late at night and keeping your area of the room neat.

★ **NOTE**: *Give your hotel number to your family and closest friends only. That's all! After a very long day of rehearsals and stress, the last thing you need is a lot of people calling your room. Though people mean well, it's best if they leave you a message, send letters, or flowers. Trust me – I speak from experience. Don't get caught up on the telephone. You will have limited time anyway, and that time needs to be spent sleeping and reviewing your index cards. Remember your goal!*

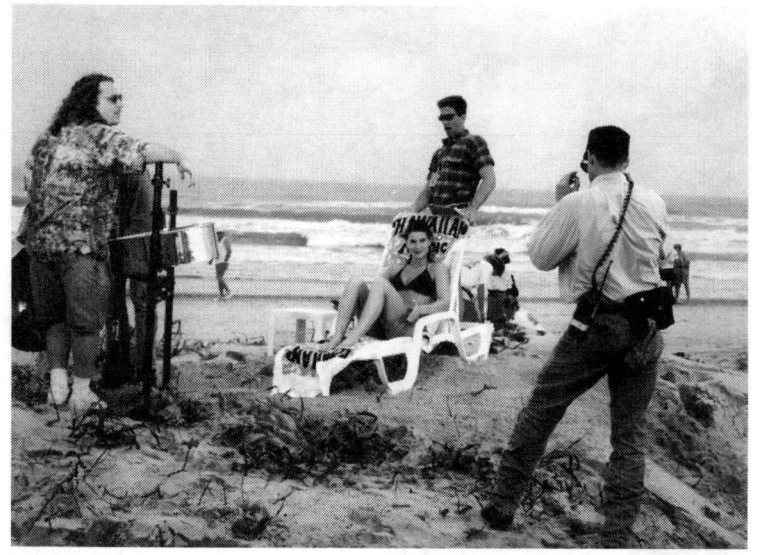

*A television crew tapes me in Jantzen swimwear
for the 1995 Miss USA® pageant.*

★ **NOTE:** *Give your address to friends, family, and co-workers. I
can't express enough how wonderful it is to receive letters, faxes, and
flowers throughout your stay. It means so much, and it gives you a
little boost.*

Rehearsals

In an effort to produce an entertaining show, all pageant productions will rehearse. Rehearsals are vital, but
they're also exhausting. It's a good idea to be fully prepared. Rehearsals seem tedious, but they're crucial. The
last thing anybody wants is for one of the delegates to look
left when she should look right. Here's a list of what to
expect during rehearsals:

★ Opening Number (Dance steps)
★ On Stage Patterns for Swimsuit/Evening gown Interview/Talent/Crowning
★ Production Number (National and International levels)
★ Top Finalists Selections
★ Judge's Questions
★ Finale

Here's a list of items you'll need to take to rehearsal:

☐ Tote bag
☐ Index cards (Study during breaks)
☐ Comfortable shoes
☐ Competition heels (Practice walking on stage during breaks)
☐ Sweater or Jacket
☐ Pillow (This isn't necessary, but rehearsals do get long. We often napped during breaks.)

★ **NOTE:** *Do not wear heels or uncomfortable shoes to rehearsals. They drain your energy.*

I was always amazed at the delegates who didn't pay attention or worse, spoke when the choreographer was explaining things. First of all, it's disrespectful. Secondly, you will miss an important piece of information that could make you look silly on stage. If you think you'll be tempted to talk or not pay attention, sit away from the group of delegates. It is a matter of concentration, not rudeness. You are there for a purpose. Even though you may get bored, sleepy, or excited, you must always remember to:

READ YOUR INDEX CARDS!

PAY ATTENTION!

STAY FOCUSED!

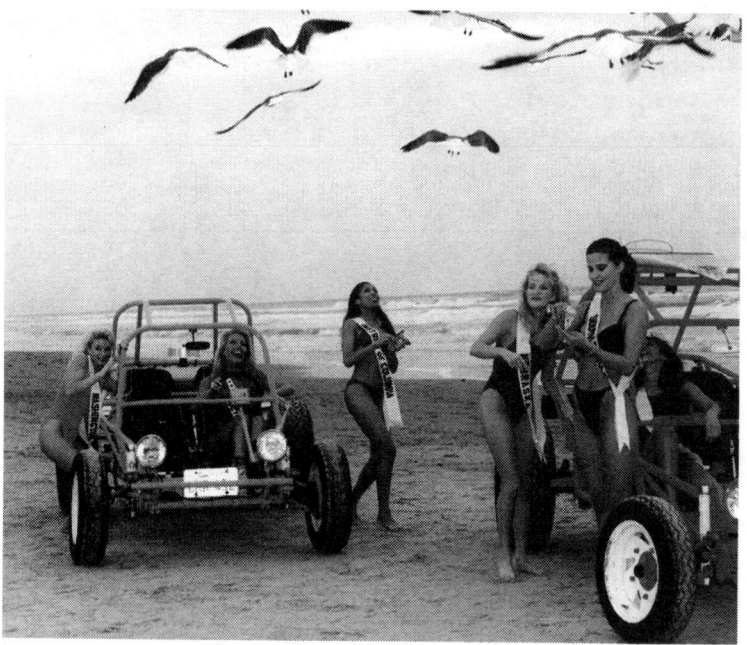

1994 Miss USA® contestants pose with birds on the beach for a promotional spot that aired during the telecast. I'm on the far right.

Dress rehearsal

Dress rehearsal usually takes place the day before or the day of the final night. It's held to make sure the production crew has everything in place for the show. Local and state pageants sometimes don't conduct dress rehearsals, but national and international competitions always do.

I realize dress rehearsals are a hassle. You wear your swimsuit and your evening gown, all in full make-up and hair. But it's a necessity, and you should take it seriously. And by the way, if the dress rehearsal doesn't get your blood pumping, then you're in the wrong place.

Chaperones

Each pageant has chaperones to accompany the delegates. These ladies are usually volunteers, and are likely to be proud of their affiliation with the pageant. The chaperone is your guardian during your stay. She travels with you, and will help answer your questions. Treat your chaperone with respect and be considerate. Don't forget to drop her a thank-you note.

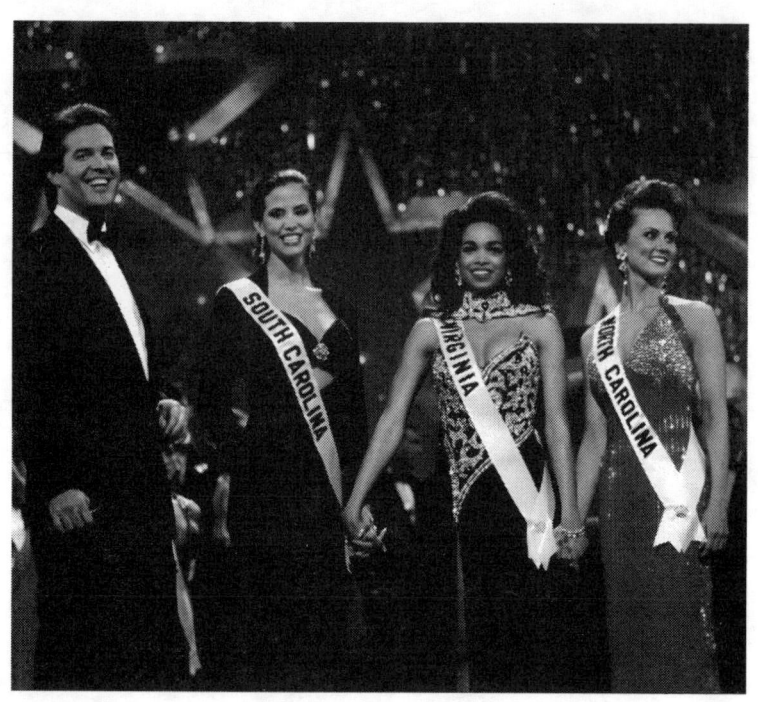

L to R: Host Bob Goen and the top three finalists at the 1994 Miss USA® pageant: Miss South Carolina (me), Miss Virginia, Pat Southall; and Miss North Carolina, Lynn Jenkins.

COMPETITION 5

"No one knows what he can do until he tries."
— LATIN PROVERB

Preliminaries

Preliminary competition is common at national and international pageants. It is less common at the state level. During the preliminaries, delegates are judged in swimsuit, evening gown, and in some cases, talent, depending on the pageant. The scores ultimately determine the top 10 or 12 finalists.

If you fail to consider preliminary night serious business, it could cost you the crown. You cannot let your guard down. Preliminary night is important, and you should respect this night as if it were final judging.

★ **NOTE:** *On the final night of competition, chances are, you'll have two to three hours to get ready backstage. Continually compliment yourself during this time. It will help you relax. I also suggest wearing headphones backstage. Bring several favorite CD's or tapes and listen to them while you get ready. It will relax you and keep you isolated from all the backstage chatter.*

Interview

The interview can be the deciding factor between winning and losing a pageant! In most cases, delegates are escorted to a judge's room for the interview. Once you're in the room and actually going through the process, the time flies. Utilize this time to your best ability! Here is a checklist to help you excel:

INTERVIEW CHECKLIST

★ Learn something about the judge's personal background so you can relate to him or her.

★ Study the judge's profile before you go in for the interview.

★ Acknowledge their talents, or career. Put this information on your index cards. (As soon as I found out who the judges were, I had my family get information on them that wasn't already in the program book. The internet is an excellent source.)

★ Take four or five deep breaths before entering the room.

★ Be natural. Laugh.

★ Shake their hand if possible during the introduction and departure. Always shake hands firmly. No one is impressed by a weak handshake.

★ Talk to a judge as you would speak to a friend. Think of them as new pals. They're probably nervous too. Make them feel comfortable.

★ Speak from you heart. Touch their heart.

★ Don't brag "me me me!" You can tell them about yourself, but don't continually pat yourself on the back.

★ Again, be honest!

★ Make eye contact often during the interview.

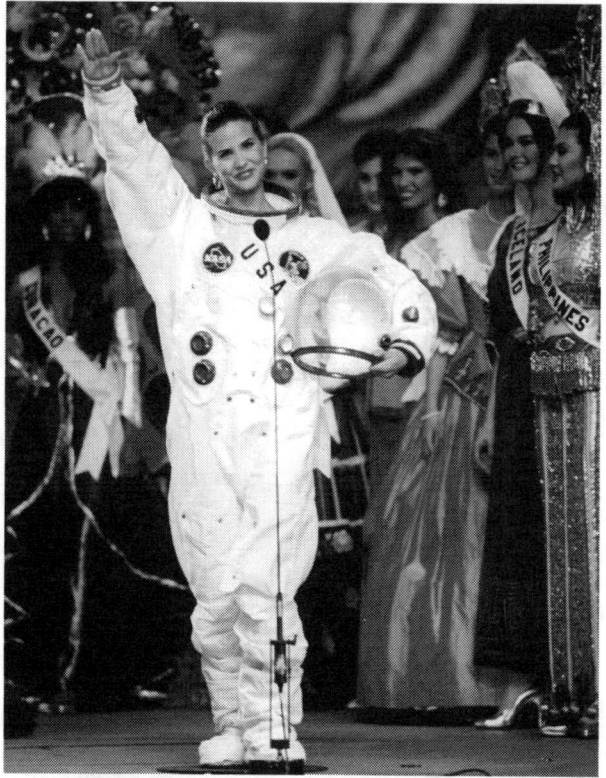

*Wearing a NASA space suit during the opening
ceremonies of the Miss Universe® pageant.*

★ If possible, say their name often during the conversation. Don't overdo it.

★ Be respectful. Be professional. Be yourself.

★ Let them know you want to be Miss_____ so you can make a difference. What will that difference be?

★ Never let the interview be a question/answer session. It should be a conversation between two new friends. Silence makes both people nervous.

★ Trust yourself.

After the interview

When the interview is over, don't stop thinking! Go somewhere quiet and analyze what was discussed in each interview. It's important not to criticize yourself. **Think Positively!** Continue to study your index cards, even after the interview. Remember, if you are chosen as a finalist, you will have more questions to answer on stage.

★ **BIG MISTAKE:** *Do not discuss your interview with the other delegates. It's inevitable the other delegates will discuss their interview with you. Don't get caught up in that situation. Be polite and walk away.*

Opening/Introduction

The opening of a pageant frequently consists of a production number which may involve a dance routine, introductions of the delegates, or both.

Swimsuit competition

The swimsuit competition isn't as difficult as some delegates believe. If you've worked faithfully on your body and you feel you look good, you do! You may be asked to walk casually in front of the judges, or

TIPS
- When speaking into the microphone, stand straight and tall. Don't lean into the microphone. It looks awkward.
- Speak up. If the audience can't hear you, neither will the judges.
- Don't overdo it. Speak clearly and soundly into the microphone without screaming. (When I introduced myself, I tried to remember to sound calm, professional, proud, and excited all at the same time. It's tricky, but with practice, you can do it correctly.)
- During rehearsals, have a friend or family member listen to your introduction.

you may have to do a front and back stance. In either case, remember to have confidence in your body. This part of competition is important, but also realize many major titleholders don't always have a perfect body.

During swimsuit competition, you should continue to show your personality. Even though you want to appear relaxed, don't walk too loosely. You must remain poised for the judges. Be sure not to swing your hips too much. When you stand to present yourself, make sure you stand at an angle to the judges. Never put your body in a direct line with the judges. It makes you look thick.

TIPS

- Never wear hose or stockings with your swimsuit even if the director says it's okay. It doesn't look good!
- Never put oil or excessive amounts of lotion on your legs. Believe it or not, these products make your legs look bigger than they are. Body builders use it to look bulky.
- Don't use products that claim to keep your swimsuit stuck to your buttocks. Find a swimsuit that fits properly. (I have seen girls use these products. When they walk on stage, their swimsuit is in place, but they also have a handprint on their buttocks. How embarrassing!)

Evening gown competition

Besides the interview, this is my favorite part of competition. The music, the atmosphere, and my gown always made me feel regal. I discussed earlier about choosing an appropriate competition gown, and now you will understand why it's so important to feel good in your gown.

During evening gown competition, you want to appear queen-like. First and foremost, think of yourself as a queen. When you're backstage getting ready to go out on stage, take

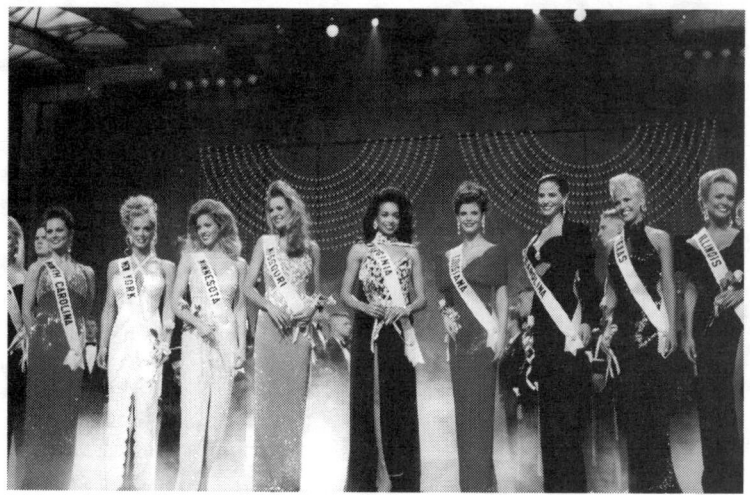

The top ten finalists of the Miss USA® pageant.
I'm third from the right.

3 to 4 slow deep breaths and listen to the music. Remind yourself how beautiful you look, and tell yourself *"The audience and judges want to see me. They're excited about me appearing on stage."* Be proud of who you are and let it show on stage. This gives you a positive aura, and it's a great way to relax.

Chances are, you'll walk an assigned pattern on stage. Every delegate will repeat the same pattern. It's important to walk at a steady pace. You don't want to rush on and off stage, but at the same time, you don't want to move so slowly that people become aware of your pace. Find a happy medium. This is your time to shine, so use it to your fullest advantage! Delegates often confuse pageant walks with runway modeling. In a pageant, you aren't showing your outfit, you are presenting yourself. The gown is an added accessory. If you have done runway modeling before, be very careful you don't fall back into the habit of "model" walking during competition. Runway models usually sway from side to side, and they use their arms more. If you walk like a runway model, your imaginary "queen crown" will fall off. There's too much swaying.

Stand tall (or at least think tall) and walk gracefully. It helped me to think of myself floating across the stage instead of walking. If you are required to turn, don't rush. And remember, always stay at an angle to the judges. Your figure will appear slimmer. You won't pick up these skills overnight, but with practice, you'll become more comfortable.

When approaching the end of the stage, **it's crucial you make eye contact again with every judge!** They are the people who take you to the next level.

Selection of finalists

This is a big moment for the delegates, the judges and the audience. It's very important you show well here! In most incidents, the previous scores are erased at this point, and the delegates are on equal footing again. Each pageant is different in the way the finalists are presented, but there are some things you should remember no matter what the format looks like.

When your number or name is read out loud, the first thing you should do is find the judges. Then walk to your appropriate spot on the stage, and again make eye contact with each judge. Thank them with your eyes, and with hand motions.

Every time I watch a pageant, I am still amazed by the different ways delegates react when their name is chosen. Some scream, some jump up and down, and I've even seen girls run to their position. It's imperative you show excitement, but at the same time, you need to remain in control. Remember to walk like a lady. Believe me, I wanted to dance when I was chosen, but I stayed focused.

When you're in the finalist's lineup, the pageant coordinators may keep you standing on stage for a few minutes. If this happens, you will be in front of the judges. Don't feel you must keep a constant smile. It's okay to relax your mouth. The judges will know if you have a fixed smile. A fake smile will look like a fake smile. As hard as it may seem, try to be natural and calm.

REVIEW

★ Be sure to thank the judges when you're called as a finalist.

★ Walk gracefully to your appropriate position. Don't run, jump, or scream.

★ Smile naturally. Don't keep a fixed smile for a long period of time. It looks unnatural.

Finalist on-stage questions

You have made it to the finals! It's time for another interview. In this part of competition, the judges are looking to see how you conduct yourself in casual conversation. I really enjoyed this part of the competition, because you have a chance to show your personality. The format usually consists of the master of ceremonies asking you familiar questions from your application. Expect questions related to what you discussed on your application such as hobbies, career, or education. Avoid being too giggly, because you may appear dense. Be polite and be yourself. If something is funny, laugh, but use good judgment. For the audience's sake, don't ramble!

Top 5 or 6 final questions

After the major competitions, the field is narrowed to the top five or six finalists. At this point of competition, stress is a major factor. If you stay calm, everything will go smoothly. The previous scores are usually erased at this point, giving the delegates an equal opportunity to advance to the next level.

★ **NOTE:** *Acknowledge and thank the judges again at this next level.*

When I was chosen as a finalist at the **Miss USA®** pageant, I felt everything happened too fast. I was numb from adrenaline. I remember thinking to myself, *"You better start getting nervous. This is it."* But you know what? The truth is, you have to remain calm, and after all you have accomplished so far, you will.

The format varies here from pageant to pageant, but in the Universe system, the judges ask the questions. You draw a number that is assigned to a judge, and then that judge asks you the question. Don't ramble! Answer it succinctly. The judges are looking for you to present your opinion in a logical way. They won't necessarily agree with you, but you should be confident with what you say.

When the judges ask you a question, they're focused on themselves at that moment. They're performing in front of the public as well. A quick, decisive answer on your part will calm their nerves.

At the Miss USA® pageant, I was asked, "If you were a member of the FCC, what would you do about shock jocks in the media?" At that time in my life, I didn't listen to morning radio, and I wasn't familiar with the term "shock jock." It was terribly scary to say the least, but I took what knowledge I did have and presented the best answer possible.

Actually, I don't even think my answer was strong, but the more I review the tape, I think the selling factor was the confidence I demonstrated in my answer. I believe the judges saw that. My point here is you can't get flustered. Take a second to think about what you will say, and then try to compose your answer the best you can. Nobody is perfect.

Top 3 final question

When you advance to this level, thank the judges again. Some pageants stop questioning at the top five/six level and choose the winner at this point. At **Miss USA,®** **Miss Teen USA,®** and at **Miss Universe,®** the top three delegates are now asked another question, the same for each contestant. Each finalist is given the opportunity to answer the same question in her own way. Use the same thoughts and tactics at this point as you did for the top five/six finalists' question.

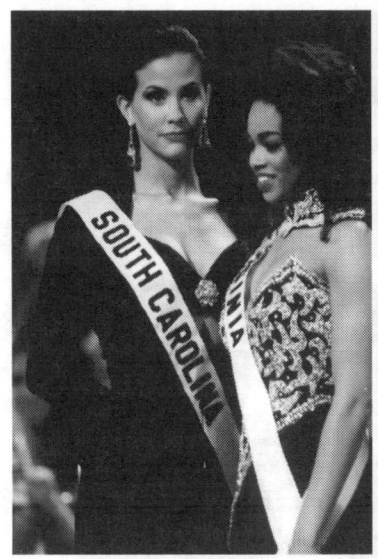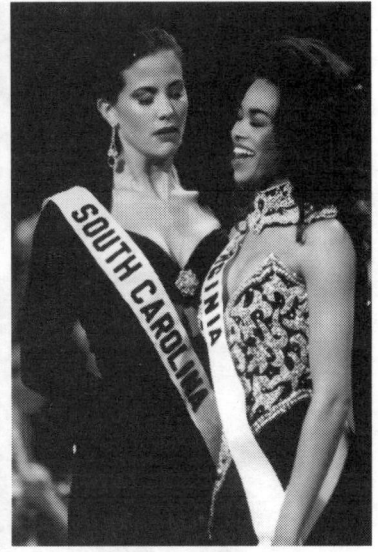

*Pat Southall, Miss Virginia, and I wait and react
as I'm announced the winner. The pictures were taken
within seconds of one another.*

The final decision

The format for most final announcements is as follows: The second runner-up is announced. Then the last two delegates are presented, and the master of ceremonies says those words we all know so well, that if for any reason the winner isn't able to complete her duties, the obligations will then be given to the first runner-up.

Catching the Crown

Hearing your name announced as the winner is like a dream! I kept thinking someone was going to say "Okay, cut! Let's do it again."

The reigning queen will usually crown and sash you

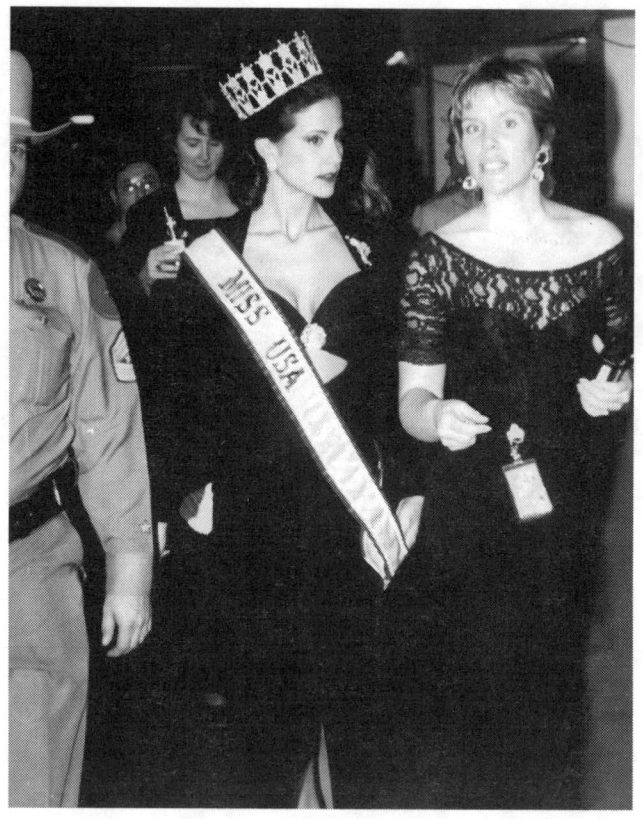

Kellie Totten, the public relations director, and I rush to the press conference minutes after I was crowned Miss USA.®

at this point. To help her out, stand as steady as possible and face forward so she can get the sash and crown placed on you properly. As I've mentioned, the first thing you should do is thank the judges for allowing this to happen.

Some people believe you shouldn't cry. Others will ask, "Why didn't you cry?" Do what feels natural. I think I was in such shock, I didn't realize what was happening. Honestly, I wanted to do a little dance, but my dress was too tight.

Directly following your crowning, there's often a photo opportunity for the press, sponsors, family, and fans. Also, depending on individual pageant directors, there's sometimes a party held for the new queen that night. The new titleholder might be asked to say a few words at the celebration. It's hard to give you advice on what to say here. I thanked everyone I could think of. Most importantly, be gracious.

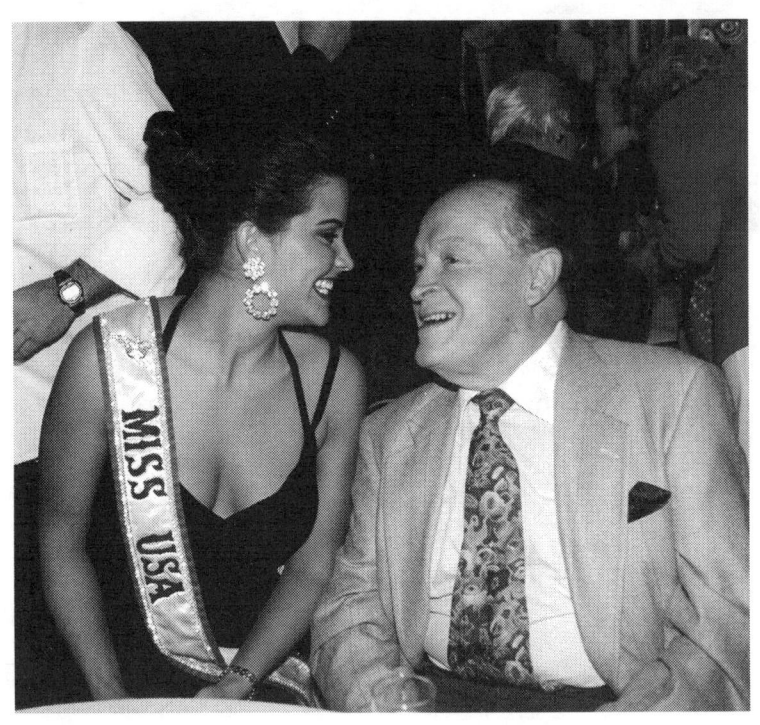

With Bob Hope at a charity event in Florida in 1994.

ROLE OF
THE QUEEN

"It matters not what you are thought to be, but what you are."
– LATIN PROVERB

Role model

When you win a pageant, you automatically become a role model for many women and children. This is perhaps the most important aspect of your reign.

There will be easy days, extremely busy days, and even some days when you may forget the importance of your position. Unfortunately, many reigning queens feel they only have to conduct themselves properly at sponsored events. Remember, someone is always watching your actions, no matter where you are or what you are doing. Without meaning to take all the fun out of life, here are some things to avoid during your reign.

AVOID

★ **Smoking:** If you must smoke, only smoke in the privacy of your room. Never smoke in public!

★ **Alcohol:** Never drink while you're working (even if you're old enough). Also, don't take a picture while holding a cup or glass of any liquid. Even if it's water, trust me, someone will assume it's liquor.

★ **Drugs:** Self-explanatory.

★ **Cursing:** EXAMPLE: *You slam a door on your thumb and you curse. Someone will remember and say, "Can you believe the mouth on Miss_____?"*

★ **Bad-Mouthing**: Don't ever bad-mouth your pageant headquarters, director, or any sponsor. If you have a problem, address the issue privately.

★ REMEMBER: *Adults and children watch and listen to you constantly throughout your reign. It's the price of winning – and it's worth it.*

You should also dress professionally. By this, I don't mean you have to wear a gown or a business suit during every minute of your reign, but be aware of what each sponsor or event coordinator is expecting of you at an event. The appropriate dress can vary from sports attire, to a casual pants outfit, to a business suit, to an evening gown. People will anticipate your arrival, and they expect you to look good.

Travel

Depending on the level of your title (local, state, national, international), you will travel. Obviously, some will travel more than others. It makes life easier if you plan ahead. (*See packing section.*) I always found it helped keep me organized if I got an itinerary from the pageant director.

Always take your sash and crown! Sometimes your crown isn't required at an appearance, but take it anyway because people (especially children) love to see it. It's also a good

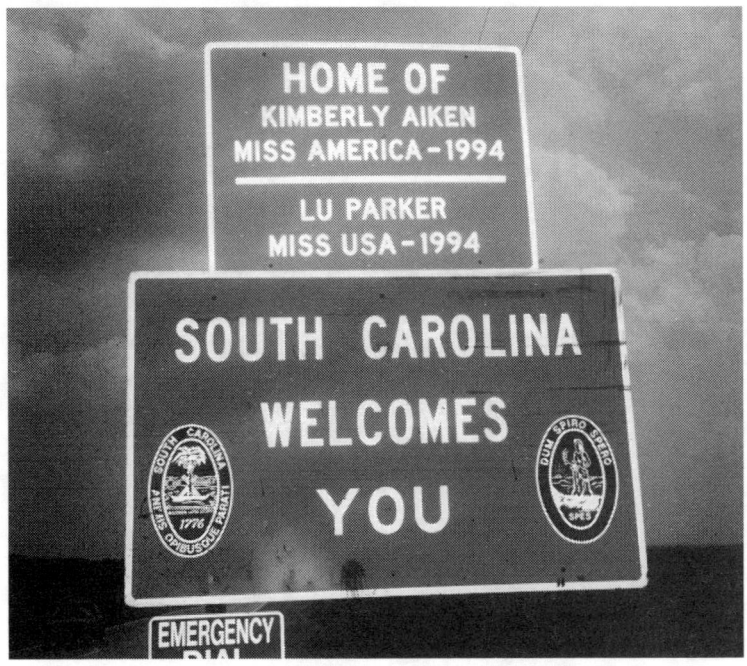

South Carolina state road signs honoring Kimberly Aiken, Miss America 1994, and Lu Parker, Miss USA 1994.®

idea to carry a camera with you when you travel. The year goes by quickly. If you don't take pictures, you may forget some wonderful experiences.

★ **NOTE:** *Carry extra publicity photos and business cards with you when you travel. I made many friends along the way, and they often asked for a picture. It's nice to have one available. It's also important to have a business card handy. Exchanging cards with people you meet could help you down the road when you need specific business connections.*

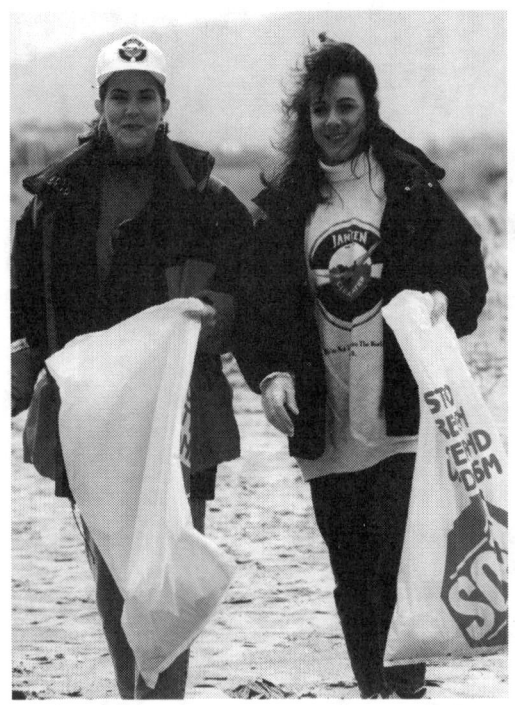

With Denise White, Miss Oregon 1994,
at a beach cleanup in Portland.

Just about everyone asks for autographs: bell captains, limo drivers, taxi drivers, and waiters/waitresses. It's fun to chat with a young child, and then surprise them with a picture and autograph.

Appearances

The appearances you make during your year will vary greatly. On one hand, this gives you an opportunity to experience many new situations and to meet interesting people. On the other hand, sometimes you may not be mentally prepared to do what's asked of you. My advice is to prepare for anything! If event coordinators tell you beforehand they don't need you to address the crowd, don't necessarily believe them, because situations often change. Always be prepared to speak. People love to hear from titleholders.

Speaking to a group of people can be easy. Address everyone in a friendly manner, and impress upon them how honored you are to be participating. If it's a charity, you can congratulate them for taking time from their busy schedule to talk about the important cause. As simple as this sounds, if you have no idea what to say, try "I hope you all are enjoying this event as much as I am."

If the sponsors give you a pre-written speech, don't get bent out of shape. Briefly look at the paper, and don't worry about saying it exactly how they've printed it. Improvise! I always reviewed the speech, and tried to remember the important parts. Then I just spoke from my heart, while incorporating what they really needed me to say. After doing it a few times, it should become second nature to you. Remember, the crowd is your friend. They want you to do well.

Dealing with the media

Throughout your reign, you will have dozens of interviews with both print and television reporters, and as you move up the pageant ladder, from local to state to national, the press coverage increases.

Reporters' questions are very different from those asked by the pageant judges. Be prepared for a wide range of char-

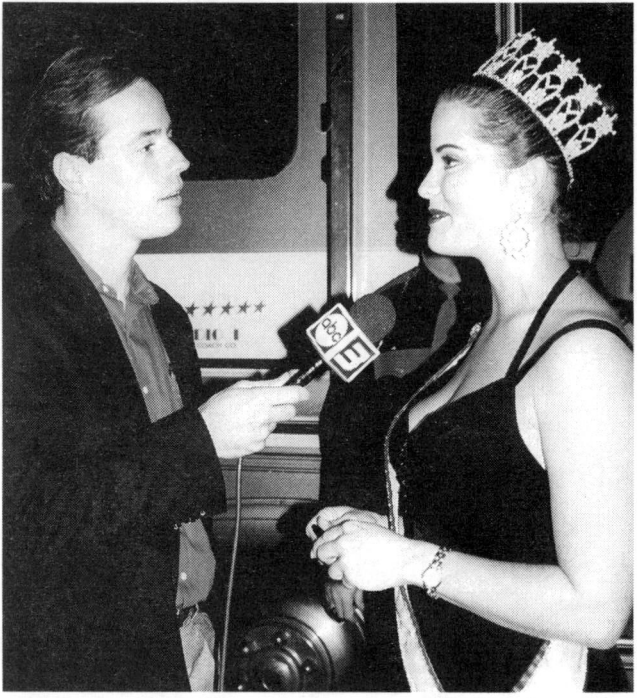

Being interviewed by a reporter at a Florida charity event.

TIPS

- Interviews should be fun. Enjoy them!
- Get to know the reporter/interviewer as soon as possible.
- Think before you answer.
- Ask yourself "What three things do I want to tell?"
- Be hospitable and friendly. Even if you don't like the line of questioning, it will be harder for them to do a negative piece if you're friendly and show them respect.

acters in the media. Some people fear the press, but you shouldn't. They help you tell your story. Again, just like the judges, they're human beings. Don't forget this point!

When I won **Miss South Carolina USA,**® I had the opportunity to do a few interviews with newspapers and television stations. But, when I won the **1994 Miss USA®** title, I was quite surprised at my next media experience. I walked into a room, and stepped up on a platform with a microphone only to look out at approximately seventy-five journalists. I was amazed! But I soon realized, this was just the beginning.

Frequently asked media questions

★ Why are you here? (Asked when you are on a specific appearance)

★ What are the responsibilities of being Miss_____?

★ How are you preparing for the State competition? National competition? International competition?

★ Describe yourself. Describe your career.

★ What do you say to people who argue pageants are degrading to women?

★ What are your beauty secrets?

★ Why did you enter the pageant? Have you always competed in pageants?

★ What do you hope to accomplish this year? What are your goals?

★ What is the difference between the USA and America pageants?

Autograph sessions

Be prepared! Beauty pageant fans absolutely love to get your autograph!

Once again, the number of signings and official autograph sessions will depend on the level of your title. Independent retailers, corporate offices, and non-profit organizations contract you for appearances. These deals are typically made through the pageant office.

The typical autograph session is harder than it may seem. If you are friendly, aware of your fan's needs, constantly signing, and are energetic, exhaustion will set in quickly.

To help, I suggest you schedule, or get the coordinator to schedule, a break for you at least every hour. It's also a good idea to have water available for you during the autograph session. It keeps you hydrated, and keeps your throat from becoming dry from constantly talking. Don't forget your breath mints.

Sometimes men will suggest you write something for a buddy. If they suggest something you don't feel comfortable writing, you don't have to comply. Don't ever feel you have to write a message that makes you uncomfortable. *Remember, it's your picture, name, and reputation.*

It's also a good idea to limit autographs to two per person. Some people will ask for more. It's not fair to the others who are patiently waiting in line. (There will always be special exceptions.)

Thank you notes

Writing thank you notes is a crucial element of a titleholder's duties *during and after* her reign. At each event, people will have invested their time and energy to make your visit memorable. You need to recognize their work.

The pageant director will often have mailing information for the sponsors. If you meet people who aren't affiliated with the event, ask for a business card. Offer your card as well. Then write where you met them, and what the circumstances were on the back of their card. This will help you personalize each note.

Throughout my year as Miss USA 1994,® I used a business card book to keep up with everyone. The book was a gift from Dayanara Torres, Miss Universe® 1993. She knew I would meet thousands of people throughout the year. Business card books can be purchased at any office supply store.

Typically, the pageant director supplies you with official stationery, but if not, use a normal card. A note takes no longer than five minutes to write and address, and it means more than you can imagine. Definitely get into the habit of writing thank you notes from day one of your preparation and continue throughout your reign.

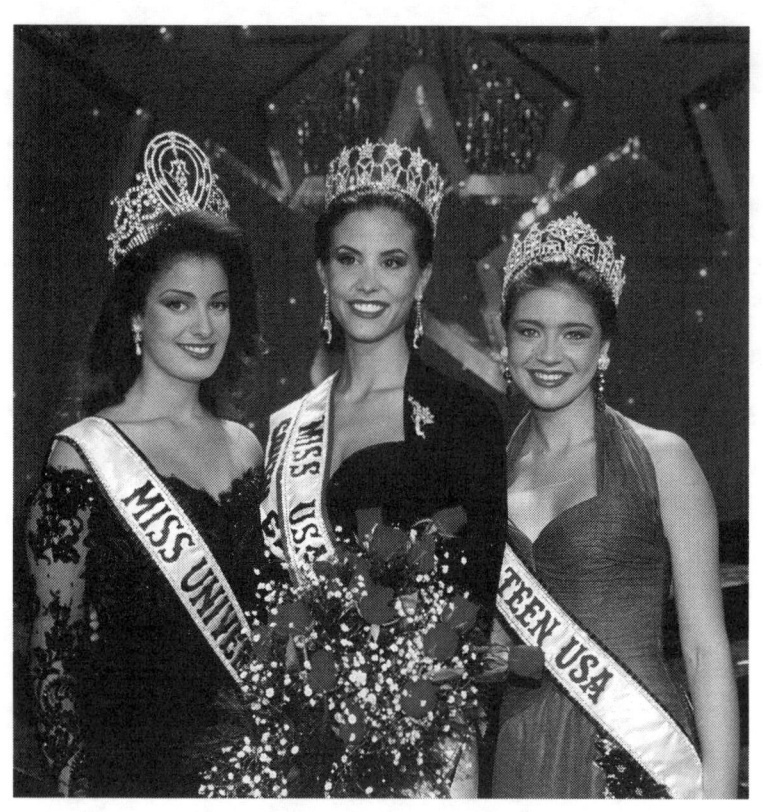

*With Dayanara Torres, Miss Universe® 1993, and
Charlotte Lopez, Miss Teen USA® 1993.*

USEFUL INFORMATION

"Uncertainty and expectation are the joys of life."
— William Congreve

Boyfriends

Winning a beauty pageant is not only an adjustment for you, but it can also be a huge adjustment for your boyfriend. First of all, you will get all kinds of attention from your friends, family, the press, directors, and naturally, other men. Of course, all of this will inevitably take time away from your boyfriend. If you have a strong trusting relationship, he should understand, and will stand by your side. But it's important to make him feel included. Sometimes we assume they know we're happy to have them around, and we forget to tell them. They need to hear us say how we feel. The best advice I can give is to ask for his patience and show some appreciation if he gives it. It doesn't mean your relationship must fail just because you win a pageant. As with any relationship, you need to work with each other to keep it strong.

Fans and fan mail

Your family and friends are usually your biggest fans, but they are hardly alone. There are hundreds of pageant fans and followers who will write to you, and follow your actions. Fans can range from young girls, to men, to women, even your own peers. I suggest dealing with them all in a similar way. Respect your position, and treat them as your backbone. Never be too busy to sign an autograph or interact with fans. Look at the opportunity as a privilege.

One of my fondest memories about fans was when I was participating in the **1994 Miss Universe**® pageant, in Manila, Philippines. The Filipinos were incredibly supportive, and were thrilled the pageant was being held in their country.

After an event, all the delegates returned to the hotel. When we arrived, a huge crowd was waiting on us. As I was being escorted through the crowd, someone yelled out my name. When I turned, there was a hand extended with something in it. I reached out and took the present as the woman called out "We love you!" The present was a silver bracelet, engraved with the words "I love you" on it. I still have the bracelet.

Fans will mail you constantly. Some letters are congratulatory, some ask for an autographed picture, while others want you as an on-going pen pal. I found if I answered a certain amount a week, the pile didn't seem so overwhelming. I suggest the same for you.

In most cases, I would simply sign a picture, and address the envelope. However, every once in a while, I read a letter that moved me emotionally, and when that happened, I would address **the fan personally** (see following letters). It is impossible **to do this with all the** letters, but remember **the fan took time out of his life** to write you. Do your best to **respond.**

Making a difference

In 1994, I visited a Juvenile Justice Center in Columbia, South Carolina. I met a number of teenagers trying to put their lives back together. Here's a letter from a boy named Lucas, and my response:

06/94

Dear Lu Parker (Miss USA),

Hey! How are things going for you? Things are pretty much the same around here. If you don't remember who I am, I was the only white, redheaded boy there. I didn't write to you at first because things were real busy around here. When you came and talked to us, for about a week I thought about you every day. There is something about you that makes me think of all the good things in life. You seem like you have a lot of love to give. You seem like a lot of fun.

Well another reason I wanted to write to you is because I'm having trouble expressing my real feelings with my parents. For the last three years I've been doing drugs and staying in trouble. Now I realize how much I have hurt my family. I'm in here for trafficking LSD. I want to tell my parents how sorry I am for what I did to them, and I want them to know that I love them. I don't know if they think I really love them. They come and visit me almost every Sunday. They bring me lots of food, clothes, whatever I need. I tell them I love them, and they tell me the same, but I'm not sure how they think I feel. If you would give me some advice on how to approach them with this that would be great. Thank you! I needed someone to tell this to and I thought of you. Well I've got to go now, but please write back and tell me what you think.

Lucas

Lucas,

I apologize for taking so long to get back to you. I am on a plane heading back to Los Angeles from a trip, and I feel I now have some time to write to you. I hope this letter finds you happy and healthy. I appreciate the kind words you wrote in your letter to me. They meant a lot! How's school? Are you keeping a positive outlook about it? I've been busy traveling, but I really have been enjoying every minute of my life. I've started acting classes, and I've decided to stay in Los Angles for at least another year.

You mentioned in your letter that you were having a hard time expressing your feelings to your family. You should never be ashamed to show how you feel. Life is too short not to communicate with the ones you love. You must realize nobody is perfect, and we all make mistakes (big and small), but that is how we learn in life. My parents always said to me when I got in trouble that it wasn't because they didn't love me, they were just disappointed in me. I used to get really upset about that statement, because as children we want to make our parents proud. Don't we? Well, you have made a mistake, but you realize your mistakes, and you are stronger because of that. Your parents love you no matter what! Take your mistake and learn what not to do in the future. Also, even though it is difficult sometimes, show your parents how much you love them. They will know you are sincere.

Remember, family is everything. You don't have to prepare to approach them with your love, just do it! Please know you are in my thoughts and prayers. Keep a smile on that cute face! Are you smiling? Smile bigger! You can do it!

Love, Lu

Remembering names

During my reign, I realized how important and how difficult it was to remember names. It's not only impressive to other people when you can remember their name, but it can make you feel more comfortable. Everything seems a bit more personal. There are many different tactics to help you remember names, and a lot of them work, but I want to share my thoughts on my "name game."

When you're introduced to someone, or when we introduce ourselves to someone, we often don't pay close attention. If we hear the name, it often doesn't register.

My suggestion is try to take the attention off you, and put it on them. Notice something about them you like, such as their smile, their eyes, or even their body. Do they remind you of someone? Then, when you hear their name, log it for a few seconds in your mind. While they are talking to your friend, or when they walk away, take their name and one characteristic about them, and make a connection to someone you know. Before you know it, you'll know the names of everyone you've met.

★ **EXAMPLE:** *I meet a guy named Tony, a guy named Ben, and a girl named Allison. How do I remember them? Easy! I say to myself, (even if they don't look like these people), "His name is Tony like my Dad." The other guy's name is Ben like my boyfriend, and the girl is Allison. She has the same quirky personality of a girl I knew in college."*

It's easy and you can add your own ideas and tactics as you experiment. Make it a habit because it really does make things a lot easier not only during your reign, but for the rest of your life. Before you know it, you'll do it without thinking twice.

Taxes

The tax man cometh! When you read the list of prizes in pageant program books, you surely don't see the tax section. But if you win prizes in a pageant, you'll have to pay a "gift tax." Just accept it from the beginning because there is no getting around it. It's especially true for state and national level pageants.

If you win a national or international level pageant, get an accountant. Don't attempt to wade through complicated tax law on your own. You might consider the same at the local and state level, depending on how much you win. At the beginning of your reign, get an estimate of how much you'll owe at tax time, so you can allot for the amount.

Prizes

Now for the good stuff. The prizes will vary depending on the pageant. I have enclosed the list of prizes I won, not to show off, but to share the great potential pageants can offer. Remember I was taxed on every single item on the prize sheet.

PRIZE SHEET FROM 1994
Courtesy Miss Universe L.P., LLLP

★ $40,000 employment contract with Miss Universe, Inc.
★ $10,000 cash and a spectacular swimwear/sportswear wardrobe from Jantzen.

★ $3,000 cash, plus an active/casual shoe collection from PayLess Shoe Source.

★ $2,000 cash, plus a complete wardrobe of !exclamation fragrance products from Coty.

★ The stunning new Miss USA Diamond Signature Brooch designed especially for Miss USA by Lauren Pipkorn for Hammerman.

★ The all-new 1994 Firebird with Formula performance package and all the upgrades, from Pontiac Division, General Motors Corporation.

★ A 1994 Cobalt Sport Boat with 175 HP Mercruiser V-6 inboard/outboard engine, convertible top, plush interior, seating for nine, swim platform, stereo system, impeccable Cobalt quality.

★ A sensational $20,000 wardrobe of evening gowns and cocktail dresses from Petals & Lace in Nashville, Tennessee.

★ An exquisite 18-karat gold and diamond Italian designed Swiss ladies watch from Bertolucci Watch Company.

★ Two Continental Airlines BusinessFirst tickets to London, Paris, Frankfurt or Madrid.

★ A $12,000 Shopping Spree of leather or fur coats and jackets, awarded by world famous Flemington Fur Company, Flemington, New Jersey.

★ A complete 35mm Maxxum SLR camera outfit, including flash, an assortment of lenses and accessories, a camcorder, plus the world's only autofocusing binoculars, and more. . . total value $10,000. . . all from Minolta Corporation.

★ An elegant wardrobe of Colesce Collection™ Lingerie and Loungewear awarded by Cameo Coutures, Dallas, Texas.

★ An extensive assortment of fashionable formal footwear by Fredereico-Leone, Colonial Shoe Company, Atlanta, Georgia.

★ A one-week "Hawaiian Vacation for Two," plus a generous supply of products from Hawaiian Tropic.

★ A personal appearance travel wardrobe and luggage from Miss Universe, Inc.

★ The beautiful Miss USA trophy.

★ The dazzling Miss USA crown from the International Gem & Jewelry Show.

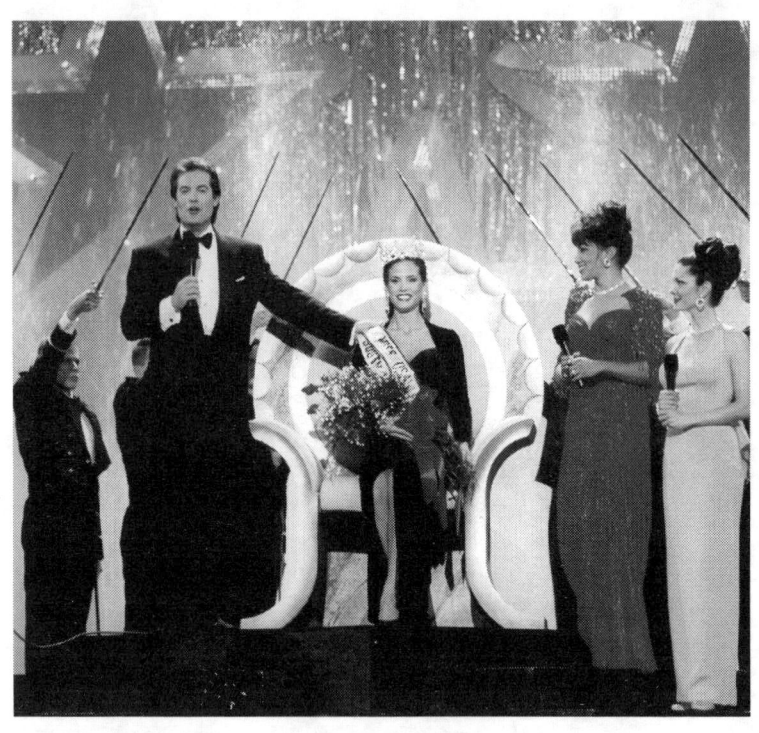

*Sitting on the Miss USA throne at the end of the telecast,
with Bob Goen and Arthelle Neville.*

RELINQUISHING
THE CROWN

> *"I came. I saw. I conquered."*
> – JULIUS CAESAR

What to expect & a few suggestions

As your year begins to come to a close, you'll likely experience mixed emotions. While some winners are often ready to give up the crown, others feel apprehensive about the future. For those of you who need some positive reinforcement during this potentially difficult time, here are a few pointers:

★ *It's been a beautiful opportunity few young women get to experience, and you've been able to live it for an entire year.*

★ *You can now use your experience in future endeavors. You've learned so much about different people, and how to interact with groups of people. It should help with anything you hope to accomplish.*

★ *All good things must come to an end, but you'll always have the memories.*

A pageant consultant once told me, *"You can't worry about giving up the crown, because once you are Miss USA, you'll always be Miss USA. It stays with you for a lifetime."*

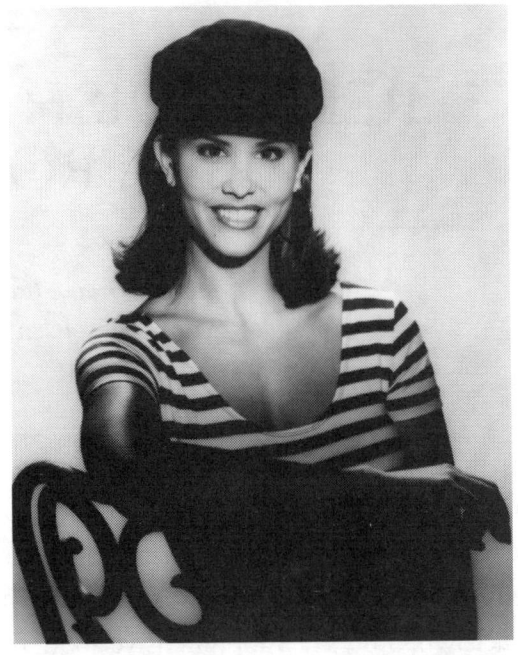

One of my promotional pictures as Miss USA® 1994.

Returning as the reigning queen is an important position. Remember, the delegates who are competing for your
title are looking to you for encouragement. You're very important in their eyes. You're where they want to be! Interact
with the delegates. Treat them in a positive way, and give
advice if they ask. You were in their position just a year ago.
Don't lose sight of that fact.

Chances are you will also be expected to give a speech
when you relinquish the crown. It's your time to share your
love and thoughts, so take time to write, re-write, edit, and
re-edit. I re-wrote my speech for the **1995 Miss USA®** pageant nearly ten times, but it was worth it.

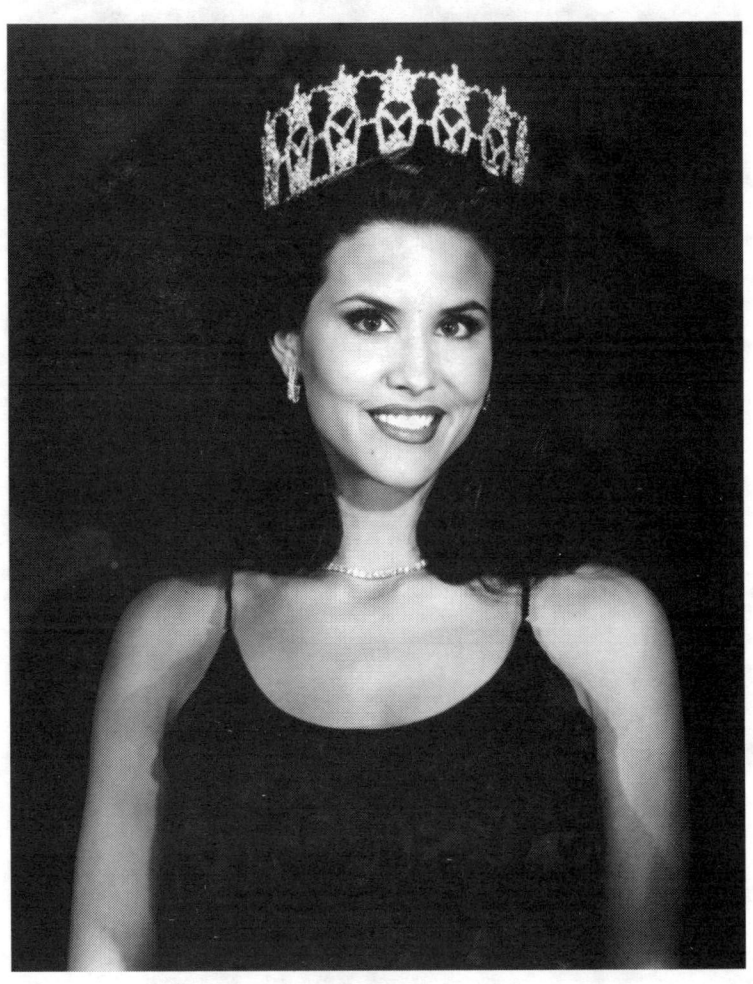

My official picture as Miss USA® 1994.

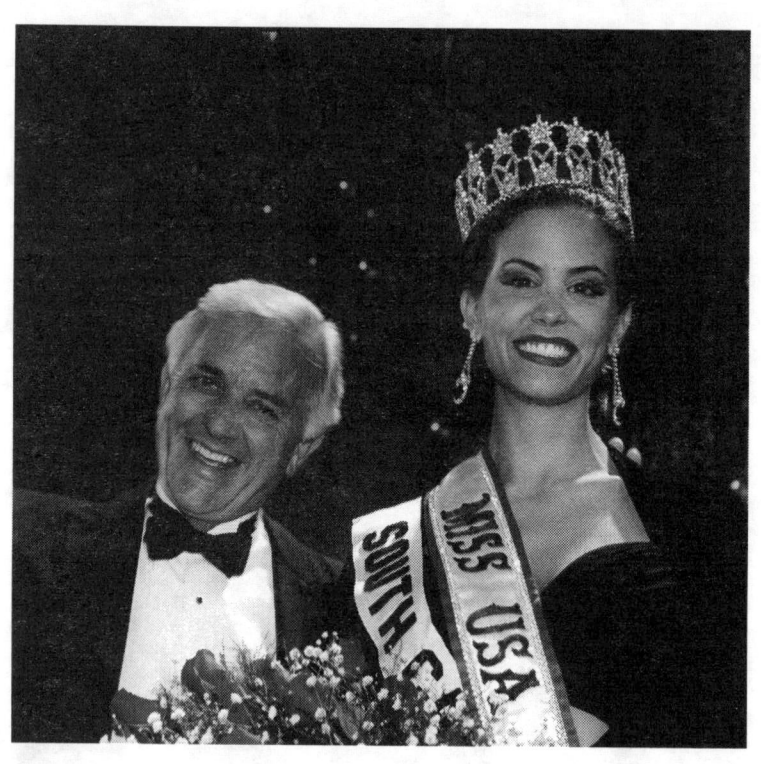

With my dad on stage, minutes after being crowned.

MY MEMORIES

"What the heart has once owned and had, it shall never lose."
– HENRY WARD BEECHER

I wrote this section to share my personal experiences during my year as **Miss South Carolina USA® 1994**, and as **MISS USA® 1994**. I also talk about competing in the **Miss Universe®** Pageant.

I won the Miss South Carolina USA pageant in December, 1993 when I was twenty-five years old. At that point, I decided to devote all my time toward preparing for the Miss USA pageant. I took a temporary leave from my high school teaching job to concentrate solely on my mental and physical goals. In between pageants, I traveled to Washington, DC to speak with officials at nine foreign embassies about the issues facing teenagers in America. It gave me the chance to interact with total strangers. I also worked daily on my physical goals, which included muscle toning and weight loss.

The mental preparation was the most challenging, and kept me busy. I read local and national newspapers every day, and developed questions and answers from the articles I read. As you might expect, I didn't have much of a social life during this time. My main focal point was the preparation for the pageant. I never lost sight of that goal.

I began writing in a journal in January, 1994. Shortly afterwards, I left Charleston, South Carolina for South Padre Island, Texas to compete in the 1994 Miss USA pageant. My journal entries at the time reflect how hard I was working to stay mentally strong. On January 30th, twelve days before the final night of the pageant, I wrote about rehearsals, swimsuit pictures, and participating in social events:

"I'm feeling strong, and I have my head on straight. It's hard at times not to break and go wild, but I am constantly reminding myself I have the 'crown' on my head."

Many of my journal entries are motivational writings I used to convince myself I was still doing okay, and to remind myself to keep a positive attitude. Throughout the first week, we went to social functions nearly every day and night, and taped segments that eventually aired on the final night, Friday, February 10th. Mainly, we rehearsed, rehearsed, and rehearsed. Often, I would go days without writing. It shows how extremely busy we must have been those last few days of rehearsals and interviews.

The last week of competition flew by for all the delegates as we anticipated those final few days, and ultimately, the final night. On Tuesday of the last week, we competed in preliminary swimsuit and evening gown. It was the first time the judges ever saw us in person. I remember being back stage waiting for the music to start for the opening number, and thinking, *"This is it. The judges are out there. I've been working months for this moment."* It was exhilarating.

Afterwards, I remember feeling good during the preliminary competition, but I also remember being emotionally low that night in my hotel room. I think it was a combination of the excitement, my anticipation of the final night, and knowing my friends and family had arrived and would be sitting in the audience. I doubted myself only once during the Miss USA pageant competition, and it was that night.

When I finally sat down with the judges, it was the highlight of the week (until the final night, of course). I felt as if I connected with each judge in a different way, and I also knew I was giving them a real sense of who I was at the time. After preliminaries, the scores were tallied. We now had to wait one more day to learn where we stood.

The energy level in the auditorium was incredible the day before and the day of competition. Not only were the delegates, staff, and chaperones there, but family members, state directors, and friends had also arrived. It was a wonderful feeling. Now we could rehearse on stage, and look out and see our family and friends in the audience. It made me feel more confident and comfortable.

The day my life changed

Friday, February 10, 1994 was the final day. We had rehearsals in the morning, then a final dress rehearsal mid-afternoon. At 5:45 P.M., we left the hotel for the auditorium, giving us two hours to get ready for the show.

It's difficult for me to explain how I felt on the actual night of the pageant. Throughout the night, from my shower to putting on my make-up to zipping up the last zipper on my opening number dress, I had an eerie feeling of awareness. I was aware of everything, and I tried to take all the good energy I felt and really experience the beauty of the moment.

Because it was a live show carried by CBS, the production had to start at a specific time. The music began; we got our cues; and all of a sudden I was walking out on the stage with a thousand thoughts going through my head. I remember feeling the excitement from the audience, and seeing the smiles on the judge's faces. I also remember looking at each judge, and thinking *"Wow! This is it!"* Of course, at the same time, I was worried about falling in my 4-inch heels. Before I knew it, I was running back stage to change quickly into a swimsuit for the announcement of the top 10 finalists.

I made top 10! After we were announced as finalists, we then had to compete in swimsuit, interview, and evening gown all over again. I was particularly nervous during swimsuit competition. When I look back at the tape, I can tell I am really uncomfortable. As the competitions progressed, I thankfully became more and more relaxed.

After I was chosen for the top six, I suddenly became surprisingly comfortable. Then a powerful thought seemed to take over my whole body. *"Lu, it's time to be nervous. You're in the top six."* But the truth is, the situation was so surreal, I was relaxed as ever.

I've already referred to the difficulty I had with my top six question: *If you were a member of the FCC, what would you do about shock jocks in the media?* My answer wasn't perfect, and I didn't say what needed to be said, but I was relaxed, and I stood behind what I was saying with conviction. I believed in my heart at this point I probably wouldn't be called to the top three. Mercifully, I was wrong. Minutes later, I was the first one called for top three. I felt like bursting out of my dress (but I wisely determined it wouldn't be appropriate).

The top three situation was comfortable for me too. I attribute much of that to Bob Goen, the host. He made me feel as if it were just the two of us on stage having a conversation instead of 300 million people watching and listening to what I had to say.

After we answered our final question, and after a television commercial break, it was time to announce the winner and runner-ups. I honestly don't remember Lynn Jenkins, Miss North Carolina being announced the second runner-up. I then remember coming back to reality when Bob asked Pat Southall, Miss Virginia and me to move forward. Just before the final announcement, I whispered something to Pat. People always ask me what I said, but I can't remember. I wish I knew. It's crazy!

When Pat and I were standing there, I didn't realize what was happening, and then I heard Miss Virginia announced as first runner-up. *"Lu Parker Miss South Carolina, you are the new MISS USA. The cash and prizes are yours, and now you can take your walk."* I didn't cry. I think I was in shock. My eyes watered when I looked out into the audience, and saw my younger brother Bill standing, flushed-faced and crying. I think only at that moment did I realize I had actually won.

After the pictures with sponsors and a press conference, I was off to the coronation ball. The celebration is a party for the delegates, their families, the judges and the pageant staff. The party seems sort of a blur to me. There were lots of hugs and congratulations. After the ball, I was escorted to my new room in the hotel. It was a generous up-grade from the room that I had been staying for two weeks. I was thrilled! I didn't go to bed until close to 2:00 A.M., and didn't sleep until after 4 A.M.

My life as Miss USA 1994

I was up at 7:45 the next morning for a photo shoot for the official **Miss USA® 1994** picture. The first thing I did when I woke up was order coffee. When it came, I naturally paid for it. Later that morning, a pageant staff member realized I had paid for room service. I remember her laughing out loud and saying, *"You're definitely the first Miss USA ever to pay for room service."* It was only the beginning of a beautiful year…all the free coffee I could drink!

The following day, I worked for Pontiac Cars most of the day shooting a commercial. I also had my first autograph session. In the evening, my friends and family had a big dinner party and reunion. The next day, I left South Padre Island for Washington DC for an appearance on *Larry King Live.*

We traveled to New York next where I made an appearance for Hammerman Jewelers, the company that designed my Miss USA diamond pendant. I also appeared on *The Jon Stewart Show* on MTV, which was incredibly cool. Then I flew directly to Los Angeles – my new home.

A few weeks later, I was off to South Carolina for an official homecoming. It was a beautiful time, and since I hadn't been back home since I left for the pageant, it was quite emotional too.

The first place I visited was North Charleston High School, where I worked before winning the state title. The school scheduled my students to come see me during their lunch break. I was filled with mixed emotions. My students were unusually quiet at first. I think it was a combination of being nervous, and the fact they had seen me on television. When they realized I was the same ol' Miss Parker, they opened up and asked all kinds of questions. When I was leaving, one of my female students hugged me and hid her face. When I asked her what was wrong, I realized she was crying. It simply broke my heart.

That same week, I spoke at the College of Charleston, where I graduated in 1990. I believe there was a person from every part of my life at the reception. I'll never forget looking out into the crowd that night, seeing people from my early childhood, from high school, and from college and graduate school. What a wonderful experience!

Before I left to go back to Los Angeles, I was able to visit Estill, South Carolina, the small town where I grew up. The town threw me a party that included local and state government officials. I was again moved emotionally because I felt so much love and support in the room. As children sang for me, I reflected on all my beautiful memories of growing up, and how fortunate I had been. It was all I could do to hold back the tears. They made March 11th "Lu Parker Day" in Estill. How cool is that?

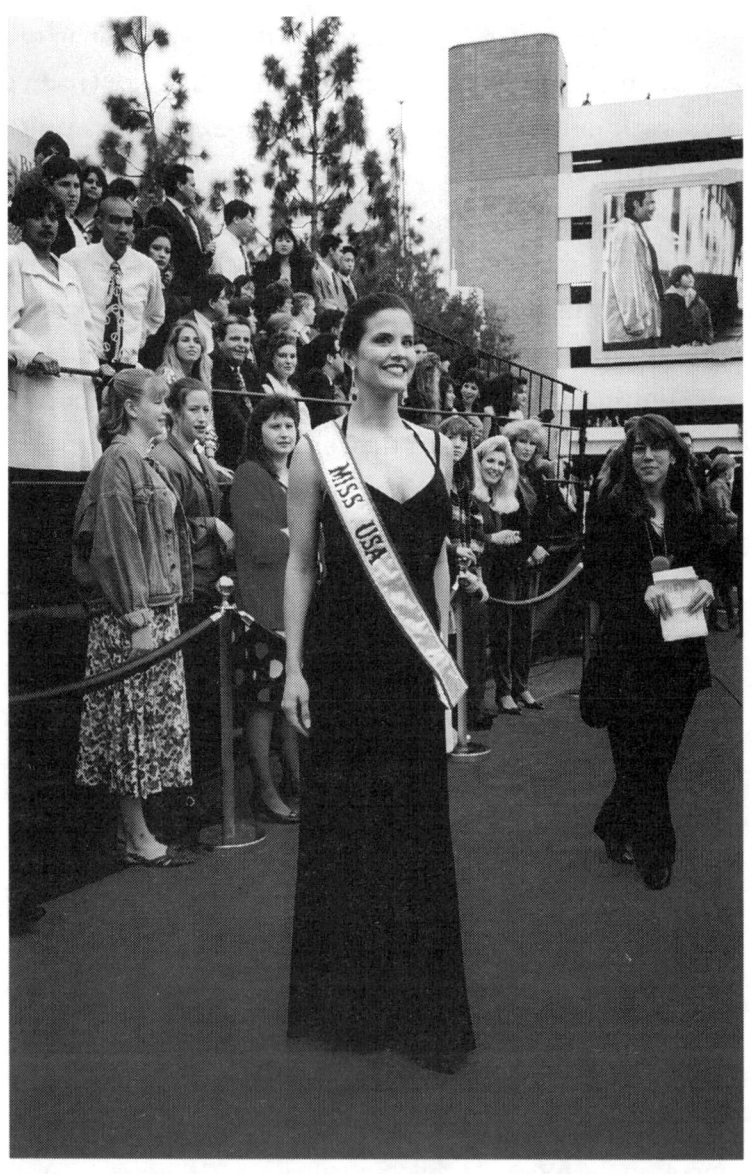

Walking on the red carpet during the opening ceremonies of the 1994 People's Choice Awards in Los Angeles.

For the rest of March and most of April, I prepared for the Miss Universe pageant, and participated in various events as Miss USA. During that time, I flew to Tennessee for fittings with the pageant gown sponsor. It was like a free shopping trip! I came home with all kinds of goodies. I also went to Austin, Texas to appear at the Miss Austin Texas USA pageant. On April 19th, I wrote in my journal:

"I can't believe it's already the 19th of April. My days have flown by so fast here. I'm also in amazement I'm getting ready to represent the USA in the Miss Universe pageant. It really just hit me."

I spent my 26th birthday in Las Vegas where I was a speaker for the Easter Seals Arthritis Telethon. I met Crystal Gayle, and Frankie Avalon. I also got to see the white tigers at the Mirage, and yes, I wasted a few quarters into those silly machines.

Competing again

On April 22, 1994, I left Los Angeles for Manila, Philippines to compete in the **Miss Universe® Pageant**. It was a difficult time for me because I didn't want to leave my family and friends, and I felt a bit isolated from the Miss Universe staff. They had become my friends, but they had to begin to remove themselves emotionally from me so they wouldn't appear to be favoring me over the other delegates. As a result, I felt a bit lonely.

When I arrived, the Filipino press interviewed me. They were very excited to be covering the pageant. After check-

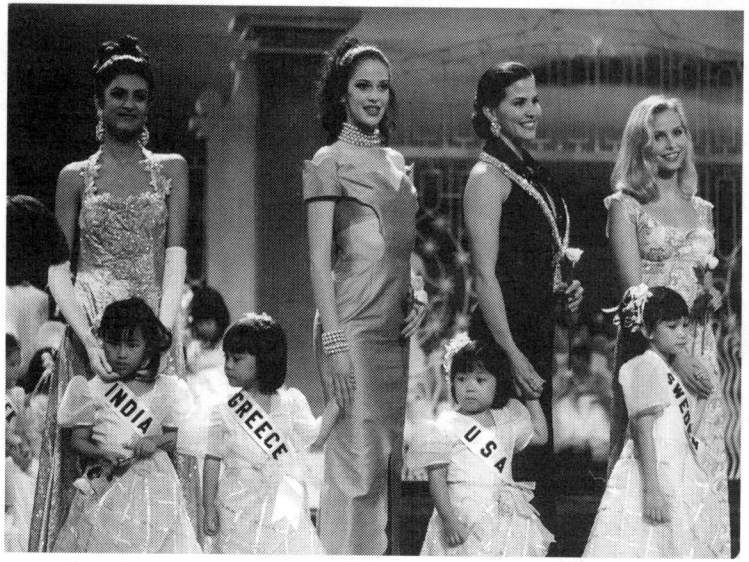

*Competing in the evening gown competition during the 1994
Miss Universe® pageant. I'm second from right.*

ing into the hotel, the next few days were filled with registration procedures, tapings, and interviews with the local
media. My roommate was Miss Sweden, Dominique
Forsberg. I was fortunate to have been paired with her because we were the same age, had similar attitudes, and connected on an emotional level. We still keep in touch.

The next four weeks in Manila were some of the busi-
est of my life. During the day we either had rehearsals, or
location tapings for the telecast. Every single night, we
dressed up and went to a social event where we were en-
tertained by Filipino guests, or by the sponsors of the pageant. The schedule was exhausting because we always had
to be "on" at the events.

Often when we were traveling back to the hotel on the buses, virtually every delegate would be sound asleep in her full-length evening gowns.

The Filipino fans were great! I was amazed at how excited they would get when we were around. I'll never forget the parade we participated in during the second week. I have never in my life seen so many people at a parade. The parade was more than five miles long, and the streets were completely covered. At some intersections, the crowds were 15 people deep. I think all the delegates enjoyed this event because it gave us a break from the monotony of social dinners and speeches. We could finally relax.

The social events and pictures continued (we must have taken at least 500, no kidding). Staying focused became increasingly difficult. The intensity of the schedule left some delegates negative and lazy. I had my moments too. Fortunately, I never expressed them in public, only when I was alone in my room.

One particular incident stands out as a real low point. One evening, I was in my hotel room on the phone, talking to people back home when a friend mentioned an Associated Press picture of me that had appeared in the newspaper back home. My friend commented about my weight and my eyebrows in the photo. Under normal circumstances, I would have blown the remarks off, but when I hung up, I simply broke down. I had never experienced frustration like that before in the pageant process.

To help with our frustrations, Dominique and I started sharing the feelings we had been hiding. It was a wonderful experience. We really bonded. Afterwards, I felt reinvigorated.

Thankfully, the days weren't all bad. There were great moments too, and no one will ever be able to experience the Philippines the way we did that April and May.

The day of final competition arrived. For the pageant to air in the United States on Friday night, we had to compete live on Saturday morning at 8 in the Philippines. (That meant a 4:00 A.M. wake-up call.) By 10:00 A.M., the new Miss Universe® 1994 had been crowned. She was the beautiful Sushmita Sen, Miss India.

I was among the top six finalists, but I failed to make it to the top 3. After being eliminated, I remember going back stage and feeling like it was all a bad dream. I wanted to cry at that moment, but something wonderful came over me. I realized I was still Miss USA, a tremendous honor. When I realized that, I felt as if ten thousand pounds of pressure had been lifted from my shoulders. I literally took my hair down, and felt like myself again. I had been focused on the pageants for so long I had nothing else to give. It was now time to relax. I had done my best, and I knew it! I could now move on and set new goals for myself. But first, I would spend some quality time with my biggest fans, my family, who had struggled through all of the preparations and competitions with me, and somehow kept me sane.

Summer

After returning to Los Angeles, I had some great experiences, and I'd like to share just a few.

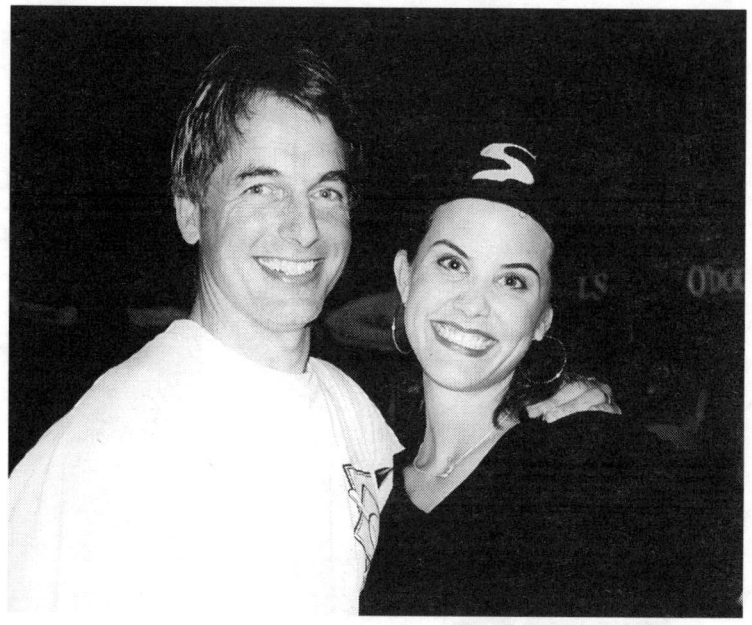

With actor Mark Harmon at a charity baseball event.

In June, I flew to South Carolina to participate in the Mark Harmon Celebrity Baseball Event. What an unbelievable trip! Not only did I get to return to South Carolina to see my family and friends, but also I made some new friends during my stay. We played in a celebrity golf tournament, visited the Children's Hospital, and played a full-fledged baseball game. To this day, I still play in the game every year. I count many of the other players among my closest friends.

One of my first Los Angeles events was a charity pool tournament at the Hollywood Athletic Club to raise money for AIDS research. Of course it was exciting for me because there were so many musicians and actors participating. We

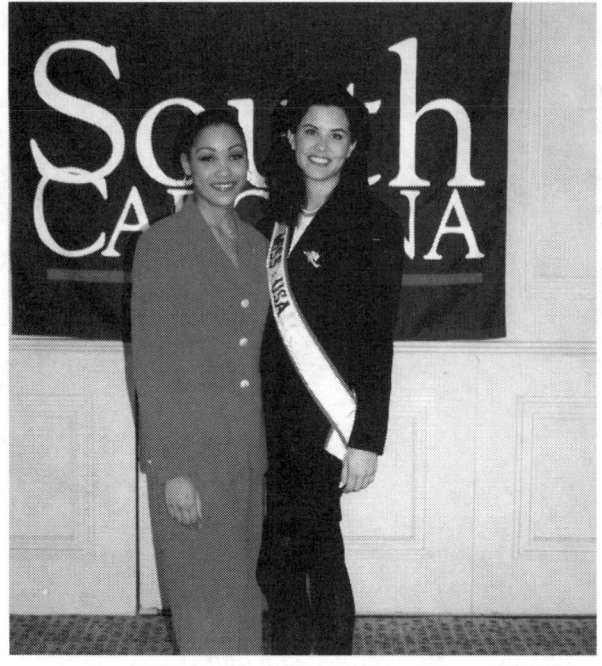

With Kimberly Aiken, Miss America 1994, in Dallas.
A couple of South Carolina girls in Texas!

won our first round (Yes, Miss USA can even shoot some stick), but we lost in the second round.

Later that month, I flew to Georgia to speak at the Alpha Delta Pi Sorority National Convention about the need for women to believe in themselves. Then I was off to Pasadena, CA to watch the USA Soccer Team play in the 1994 World Cup.

In August, after attending the 1994 Miss Teen USA® pageant in Mississippi, I caught a plane for Charleston, South Carolina. I always loved going home. This trip was for a charity fishing tournament. My family and the local CBS television crew met me at the airport. The next day, I was at the docks ready to board a fishing boat at 5:45 A. M. Ouch! The event was a Marlin fishing tournament, so, of course, I caught 3 sharks. No prizes for me. Afterwards, I hosted the party and awards ceremony.

Fall

In October, one of my fantasies came true! I was asked to be a contestant on the game show *Family Feud*. It was really cool! The theme of the show was Beauty vs. Brawn. The Beauty team consisted of Angela Visser, Miss Universe® 1989, Porntip Nakhirunkanok, Miss Universe® 1988, Christy Fichtner, Miss USA 1986,® and me. The Brawn team was "The Incredible Hulk" Lou Ferrigno, Franco Comacho, Frank Zane, and Lee Gainey, who are all former Mr. Universes. We beat them three times and they beat us twice. It's always nice to beat the boys.

Later that month, I participated in a charity event with Bob Hope in Fort Walton Beach, Florida. What an honor it was to meet Mr. Hope and his lovely wife Delores! You don't ever forget meeting a legend like Bob Hope.

My appearance later in the year on *Leeza* turned out to be particularly important for me. I realized how much I enjoyed people and how comfortable I felt in front of a camera. It was at this time that I started to begin seriously thinking about a career in television.

In early January, I began preparing for the 1995 Miss USA® pageant. It was hard to realize I'd soon be leaving my apartment and my live-in manager, but I also looked forward to the freedom of being on my own again.

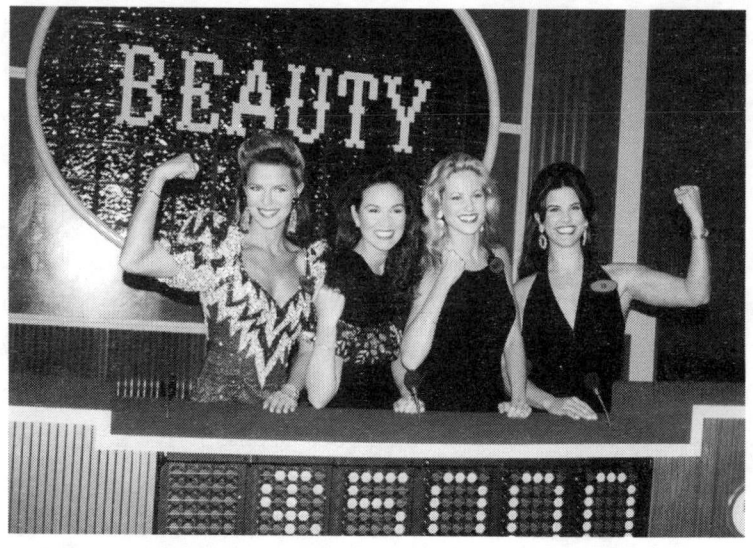

Competing on Family Feud *with Miss USA® 1986,*
Christy Fichtner; Miss Universe® 1988, Portnip
Nakhirunkkanok; and Miss Universe® 1989, Angela Visser.

Giving it up

On January 24th, I left for South Padre Island, Texas, home of the 1995 Miss USA pageant. As you might expect, it was odd going back as Miss USA rather than as Miss South Carolina USA. Less pressure, to be sure. I knew all the local volunteers, and I was definitely treated on a different level now. I must say it was awfully nice.

Because the reigning queen has to tape various segments for the broadcast, I arrived a week prior to any of the delegates. I stayed in a beautiful oceanfront suite, and I worked long hours taping for the telecast

I was there for approximately 3 weeks doing appearances, tapings, and interviews. I realize now how fortunate I was to feel the way I did at the time. I'm sure some winners have mixed emotions about giving up the crown, but I felt just right about the whole situation. As the days grew closer and closer to the final night, I felt a bit nostalgic, but also anxious to move on with my life. On February 10, 1995 I crowned Chelsi Smith of Texas as Miss USA® 1995.

As I took my final walk, it was thrilling to look out into the crowd and see all my old and new friends. I can't imagine not having those memories. The night was filled with good friends and good times. The next day, I returned to Los Angeles to begin a new chapter; one which is still unfolding today and one made richer by the years I spent challenging myself in pageants.

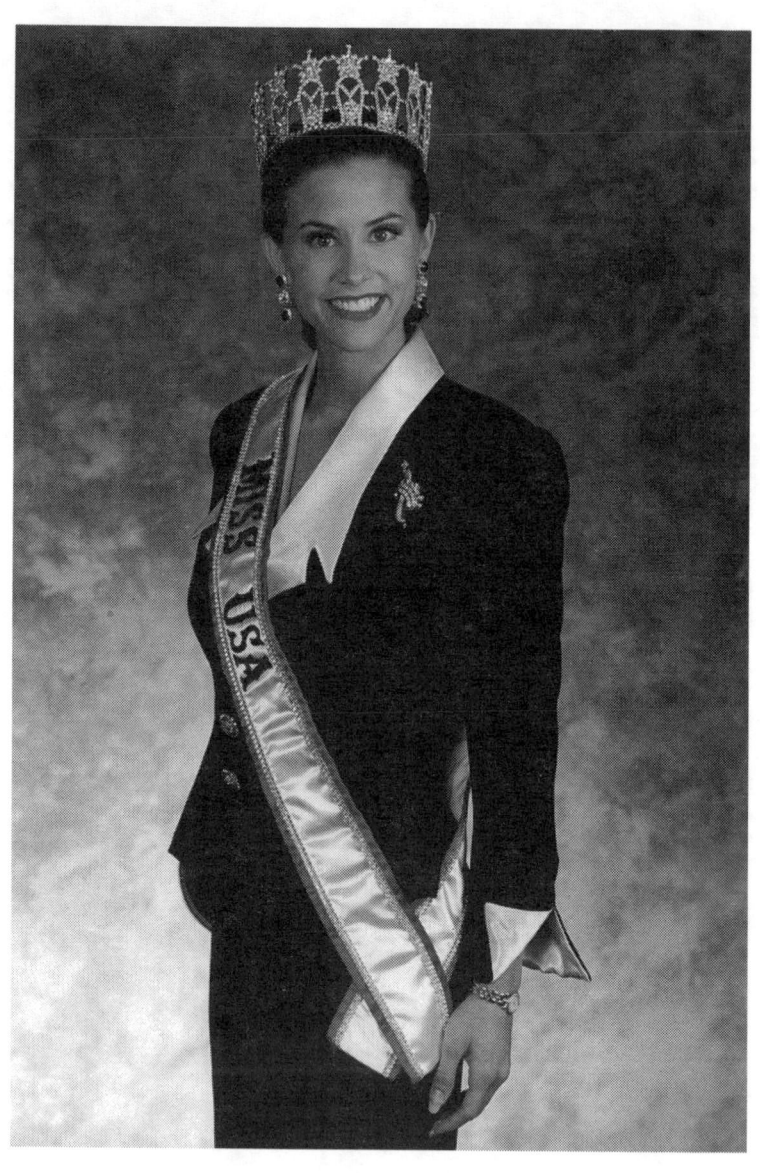

*My first official picture as Miss USA,® taken
the morning after the pageant . . . on three hours sleep!*

HISTORY OF
THE PAGEANTS

"Hitch your wagon to a star."
– Emerson

History of the pageants
Courtesy Miss Universe L.P., LLLP

Donald J. Trump and CBS purchased the Miss Universe Organization in 1997. The newly formed company is committed to producing the Miss UNIVERSE,® Miss USA,® and Miss TEEN USA® pageants with new definition, leadership, and vision.

The internationally recognized Miss UNIVERSE,® Miss USA,® and Miss TEEN USA® pageants air as live specials on the CBS Television Network, and consistently rank among the most-watched television programming in the world.

2001 will mark the 50th anniversary of the MISS UNIVERSE® and MISS USA® Pageants, which began in 1952 as concurrent events in Long Beach, California. The pageants moved to Miami Beach, Florida in 1960 and the broadcast tradition began on CBS. In 1965, the two pageants became separate live television specials, and since 1972 have been telecast from exotic locations around the globe.

Miss Teen USA®

The MISS TEEN USA® Pageant debuted in August 1983 in Lakeland, Florida, and is the premier pageant for teenage women. Since its inception, the pageant has traveled to exciting U.S. cities.

> Memphis, Tennessee (1984)
>
> Miami, Florida (1985)
>
> Daytona Beach, Florida (1986)
>
> El Paso, Texas (1987)
>
> San Bernadino, California (1988-1989)
>
> Mississippi Gulf Coast (1990-94)
>
> Wichita, Kansas (1995)
>
> Las Cruces, New Mexico (1996)
>
> South Padre Island, Texas (1997)
>
> Shreveport-Bossier, Louisiana (1998, 1999, 2000)

An estimated 200 million viewers in approximately 24 countries watch the pageant each year.

Miss USA®

Since the MISS USA Pageant began in 1952, forty-eight Miss USA titleholders, and thousands of women have contributed to making the MISS USA® Pageant a national tradition. In 1972, the 21st annual MISS USA® Pageant was held in Puerto Rico and was broadcast live via satellite for the first time. Since then, the pageant has traveled to diverse American cities, including:

New York City, New York (1973)
Niagara Falls, New York (1974-1976)
Charleston, South Carolina (1977-78)
Mississippi Gulf Coast (1979-1982)
Knoxville, Tennessee (1983)
Lakeland, Florida (1984-85)
Miami, Florida (1986)
Albuquerque, New Mexico (1987)
El Paso, Texas (1988)
Mobile, Alabama (1989)
Wichita, Kansas (1990-93)
South Padre Island, Texas (1994-96)
Shreveport-Bossier, Louisiana (1997, 1998)
Branson, Missouri (1999, 2000)

Each year an estimated 300 million viewers in approximately 30 countries tune in to watch the Miss USA® Pageant.

Miss Universe®

Satellite developments in the 1970s allowed the MISS UNIVERSE® Pageant to travel outside the United States, and in 1972, the pageant was telecast live, via satellite, for the first time from the Cerromar Beach Hotel in Dorado, Puerto Rico. From Puerto Rico, the pageant traveled to these exciting locations:

Athens, Greece (1973)
Manila, Philippines (1974)
El Salvador (1975)
Hong Kong (1976)
The Dominican Republic (1977)

Acapulco, Mexico (1978)
Perth, Australia (1979)
Seoul, South Korea (1980)
New York, New York (1981)
Lima, Peru (1982)
St. Louis, Missouri (1983)
Miami, Florida (1984, 1985)
Panama City, Panama (1986)
Singapore (1987)
Taipei, Taiwan, The Republic of China (1988)
Cancun, Mexico (1989)
Los Angeles, California (1990)
Las Vegas, Nevada (1991)
Bangkok, Thailand (1992)
Mexico City, Mexico (1993)
Manila, Philippines (1994)
Windhoek, Namibia (1995)
Las Vegas, Nevada (1996)
Miami Beach, Florida (1997)
Honolulu, Hawaii (1998)
Trinidad & Tobago (1999)
Cyprus (2000)

600 million viewers in approximately 60 countries share each year in the glamour and excitement of this live international telecast.

Miss America

Courtesy of The Miss America Organization

Rich in history and social significance, the Miss America Organization is a not-for-profit corporation that has maintained a tradition for many decades of empowering American women to achieve their personal and professional goals, while providing a forum in which to express their opinions, talent and intelligence.

The competition was founded in 1921 as a "bathing beauty" contest to extend the summer tourist season one week beyond Labor Day. Today, the Miss America Pageant is held each year on the second Saturday evening following Labor Day, with contestants gathering for the competition and rehearsals two weeks preceding the national telecast.

The Miss America competition exists for the purpose of providing personal and professional opportunities for young American women and promoting their voice in culture, politics and the community.

In addition to conducting the annual national competition, the organization acts year-round as the nation's leading achievement program and largest scholarship fund for American women.

In 1954, the Miss America Pageant was broadcast live for the very first time. That broadcast broke records of the day with 39 percent of the television audience (27 million viewers) viewing the Miss America telecast. It's broadcast each year from Atlantic City, New Jersey.

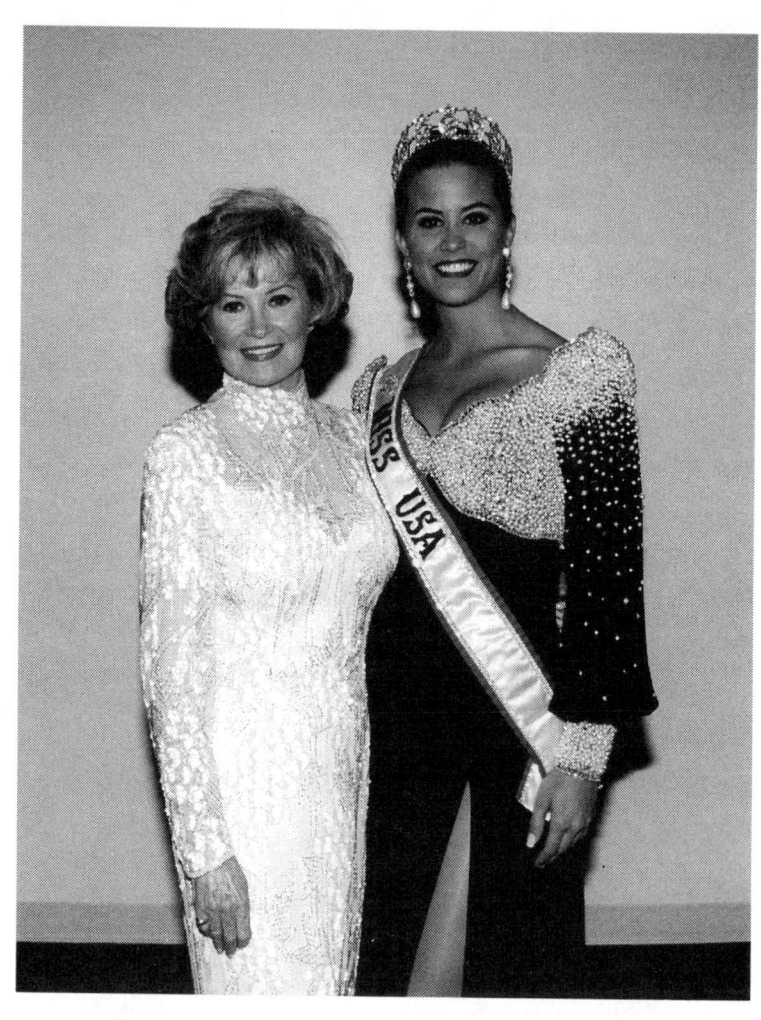

*With Jackie Loughery, Miss USA® 1952, at the
1995 Miss USA® pageant.*

PAST TITLEHOLDERS 11

"First say to yourself what you would be;
and then do what you have to do."
— EPICTETUS

Courtesy Miss Universe L.P., LLLP

Miss Teen USA®

1983	Ruth Zakarian – New York	1992	Jamie Solinger – Iowa
1984	Cherise Haugen – Illinois	1993	Charlotte Lopez – Vermont
1985	Kelly Hu – Hawaii	1994	Shauna Gambill – California
1986	Allison Brown – Oklahoma	1995	Keylee Sue Sanders – Kansas
1987	Kristi Addis – Mississippi	1996	Christie Woods – Texas
1988	Mindy Duncan – Oregon	1997	Shelly Moore – Tennessee
1989	Brandi Sherwood – Idaho	1998	VanessaMinnillo – South Carolina
1990	Bridgette Wilson – Oregon		
1991	Janel Bishop – New Hampshire	1999	Ashley M. Coleman – Delaware

Miss USA®

1952	Jackie Loughery – New York	1977	Kimberly Tomes – Texas
1953	Myrna Hansen – Illinois	1978	Judy Anderson – Hawaii
1954	Miriam Stevenson – South Carolina*	1979	Mary T. Friel – New York
1955	Carlene King Johnson – Vermont	1980	Jineane Ford – Arizona (Succeeded Shawn Wheatherly)
1956	Carol Morris – Iowa	1981	Kim Seelbrede – Ohio
1957	Charlotte Sheffield – Utah	1982	Terri Utley – Arkansas
1958	Eurlyne Howell – Louisiana	1983	Julie Hayek – California
1959	Terry L. Hutingdon – California	1984	Mia Shanley – New Mexico
1960	Linda Bement – Utah*	1985	Laura Herring – Texas
1961	Sharon Brown – Louisiana	1986	Christy Fichtner – Texas
1962	Macel Wilson – Hawaii	1987	Michelle Royer – Texas
1963	Marite Ozers – Illinois	1988	Courtney Gibbs – Texas
1964	Bobbie Johnso – DC	1989	Gretchen Polhemus – Texas
1965	Sue Downey – Ohio	1990	Carole Gist – Michigan
1966	Maria Remenyi – California	1991	Kelli McCarty – Kansas
1967	Sylvia L. Hitchcock* – Alabama	1992	Shannon Marketic – California
1968	Dorothy Anstett – Washington	1993	Kenya Moore – Michigan
1969	Wendy Dascomb – Virginia	1994	Lu Parker – South Carolina
1970	Debbie Shelton – Virginia	1995	Shanna Moakler – New York (Succeeded Chelsi Smith)
1971	Michele McDonald – Pennsylvania	1996	Ali Landry – Louisiana
1972	Tanya Wilson – Hawaii	1997	Brandi Sherwood – Idaho
1973	Amanda Jones – Illinois	1998	Shawnae Jebbia – Massachusetts
1974	Karen Morrison – Illinois	1999	Kimberly Ann Pressler – New York
1975	Summer Bartholomew – California	2000	Lynnette Cole – Tennessee
1976	Barbara Peterson – Minnesota		

---

* Became Miss Universe

Miss Universe®

1952	Armi Kuusela – Finland	1978	Margaret Gardiner – South Africa
1953	Christiane Martel – France	1979	Maritza Sayalero – Venezuela
1954	Miriam Stevenso – USA	1980	Shawn Weatherly – USA
1955	Hellevi Rombin – Sweden	1981	Irene Saez – Venezuela
1956	Carol Morris – USA	1982	Karen Baldwin – Canada
1957	Gladys Zender – Peru	1983	Lorraine Downes – New Zealand
1958	Luz Marina Zuluaga – Columbia	1984	Yvonne Ryding – Sweden
1959	Akiko Kojima – Japan	1985	Deborah Carthy-Deu – Puerto Rico
1960	Linda Bement – USA –	1986	Barbara Palacios Teyde – Venezuela
1961	Marlene Schmidt – Germany	1987	Cecilia Bolocco – Chile
1962	Norma Nolan – Argentina	1988	Porntip Nakhirunkanok – Thailand
1963	Ieda Maria Vargas – Brazil	1989	Angela Visser – Holland
1964	Corinna Tsopei – Greece	1990	Mona Grudt – Norway
1965	Apasra Hongsakula – Thailand	1991	Lupita Jones – Mexico
1966	Margareta Arvidsson – Sweden	1992	Michelle McLean – Namibia
1967	Sylvia Hitchcock – USA	1993	Dayanara Torres – Puerto Rico
1968	Martha Vasconcellos – Brazil	1994	Sushmita Sen – India
1969	Gloria Diaz – Philippines	1995	Chelsi Smith – USA
1970	Marisol Malaret – Puerto Rico	1996	Alicia Machado – Venezuela
1971	Georgia Risk – Lebanon	1997	Brook Lee – USA
1972	Kerry Anne Wells – Australia	1998	Wendy Fitzwilliam – Trinidad and Tobago
1973	Margarita Moran – Philippines	1999	Mpule Kwelagobe – Botswana
1974	Amparo Munoz – Spain	2000	Lara Dutta – India
1975	Anne Marie Pohtamo – Finland		
1976	Rina Messinger – Israel		
1977	Janelle Commissiong – Trinidad and Tobago		

Miss America

1959	Mary Ann Mobley – Mississippi		1982	Elizabeth Ward – Arkansas
1960	Lynda Lee Mead-Mississippi		1983	Debra Sue Maffett – California
1961	Nacy Fleming – Michigan		1984	Vannessa Williams – New York (Resigned)
1962	Maria Beale Fletcher-North Carolina			Suzette Charles – New Jersey
1963	Jacquelyn Jeanne Mayer – Ohio		1985	Sharlene Wells – Utah
1964	Donna Azum – Arkansas		1986	Susan Diane Akin – Mississippi
1965	Vonda Kay Van Dyke-Arizona		1987	Kellye Cash – Tennessee
1966	Deborah Irene Bryant – Kansas		1988	Kaye Lani Rae Rafko – Michigan
1967	Jane Anne Jayroe – Oklahoma		1989	Gretchen Carlson – Minnesota
1968	Debra Dene Barnes – Kansas		1990	Debbye Turner – Missouri
1969	Judith Anne "Judi" Ford – Illinois		1991	Marjorie Judith Vincent – Illinois
1970	Pamela Eldred – Michigan		1992	Carolyn Suzanne Sapp-Hawaii
1971	Phyllis George – Texas		1993	Leanza Cornett – Florida
1972	Laurel Lea Schaefer – Ohio		1994	Kimberly Clarice Aiken – South Carolina
1973	Terry Meeuwsen – Wisconsin		1995	Heather Leigh Whitestone – Alabama
1974	Rebecca Ann King – Colorado			
1975	Shriley Cothran – Texas		1996	Shawntel Smith – Oklahoma
1976	Tawny Godin – New York		1997	Tara Dawn Holland – Kansas
1977	Dorothy Benham – Minnesota		1998	Katherine Shindle – Illinois
1978	Susan Perkins – Ohio		1999	Nicole Johnson – Virginia
1979	Kylene Barker – Virginia		2000	Heather Renee French – Kentucky
1980	Cheryl Prewitt – Mississippi			
1981	Susan Powell – Oklahoma			

Pageant contacts

MISS UNIVERSE L.P., LLLP

Owner of Miss Teen USA,® Miss USA,® and Miss Universe®

1370 Avenue of the Americas
16th Floor
New York, New York 10019
Telephone: 212-373-4999

WEBSITES:
www.missuniverse.com
www.missusa.com
www.missteenusa.com

MISS AMERICA
Two Ocean Way, Suite 1000
Atlantic City, New Jersey 08401
Telephone: 609-345-7571
Fax: 609-347-6079

Website: www.missamerica.com

ABOUT THE AUTHOR

A ninth grade English literature teacher when she was crowned **Miss USA** 1994, Lu Parker became just the third South Carolinian to capture the Miss USA title. Lu went on to represent the United States in the **Miss Universe** pageant in Manila, Philippines, where she placed among the top 6 finalists. She relinquished her crown in February 1995.

Lu holds a **Bachelor of Arts Degree** in English from the College of Charleston and a **Master of Arts Degree** in Education from The Citadel.

Lu participates annually in the **Mark Harmon** Celebrity Baseball Event and in the **Louise Mandrell** Celebrity Sporting Clays Shoot. Always handy with a shotgun, Lu has taken top overall female five years in a row. In 1996, Lu carried the Olympic torch through Georgia as part of the Summer Olympics.

From 1996 to 1998, Lu worked as a news reporter at WCSC, the CBS affiliate in Charleston, South Carolina. She now works at KABB, the Fox affiliate in San Antonio, Texas, where she anchors the station's nightly newscast.

ORDER FORM

CATCHING THE CROWN
The Source for Pageant Competition

☐ Yes, I would like to order a copy of **CATCHING THE CROWN.**

Name _____

Address _____

City_____

State _____ **Zip** _____

Phone (_____ **)** _____

E-mail _____

_____ book(s) @ $19.99 + $4.00 shipping and handling each. (Add only $1 shipping for additional books.)

_____ TEXAS residents add 7.75% tax for each book.

GRAND TOTAL: $_____

☐ Enclosed is my check or money order.

Make check payable to **Parker Productions.**
Send payment to **P.O. Box 6921, San Antonio, Texas 78209.**

Please allow 7 to 10 days for delivery.